Reflexology:
A Practical Approach, Second Edition

Reflexology

A Practical Approach

Second Edition

Vicki Pitman

with Kay MacKenzie

 Nelson Thornes

First published in 1997 by:
Stanley Thornes (Publishers) Ltd

Second edition 2002 published by:
Nelson Thornes Ltd
Delta Place
27 Bath Road
CHELTENHAM
GL53 7TH
United Kingdom

08 / 10 9 8

A catalogue record for this book is available from the British Library.

ISBN 978 0 7487 6577 5

Illustrations by Angela Lumley
Page make-up by Florence Production Ltd, Stoodleigh, Devon

Printed and bound in The Netherlands by Wilco

CONTENTS

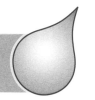

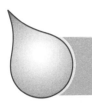

ACKNOWLEDGEMENTS

Chapter Fourteen, *Communication and understanding your client*, has been contributed by Kay MacKenzie.

I would like to express my gratitude and appreciation to the following colleagues: first, to my teacher Farida Sharan who originally inspired me to enter the field of holistic medicine and made it possible for me to take up the study of Reflexology. Next, to Allen Parrott and Kay MacKenzie who believed in me as a teacher and had the vision to offer a professional training course. Finally to Hazel Goodwin who gave much-valued support in the preparation of this book, and to John Tindall.

The IIR foot chart on page xxi is reproduced by kind permission of Dwight C Byers, President of the International Institute of Reflexology, 5650 First Avenue North, PO Box 12642, St Petersburg, Florida 33733-2642 USA. The Institute's UK address is: The International Institute of Reflexology (UK), 32 Priory Road, Portbury, Bristol BS20 9TH; tel/fax 01275 373359. The foot chart on page xxii by Chris Stormer is reproduced by kind permission of the Reflexology Academy of Southern Africa. Chris Stormer, founder and president of the Academy, can be contacted via PO Box 1280, Rivonia 2128, Gauteng, Republic of South Africa. We are grateful to Loretta Cusworth for her help in obtaining the chart. We would like to thank Kristine Walker of the Kristine Walker School of Reflexology, Brighton, for permission to use the hand charts on page 168. We would also like to thank Martine Faure-Alderson and Association Reflex Therapy Total, East Molesey, Surrey, for permission to use additional material from their work. We would also like to acknowledge the help of the staff of *Reflexions* and at Print King in providing the illustration on page xxiv and Richard Alton for the cover photograph.

INTRODUCING REFLEXOLOGY

As students training in professional reflexology you may already have a general idea about what reflexology is. At one time the term 'reflexology' was almost entirely unknown to the general public but this situation has largely changed in recent years and today more and more people have heard about reflexology but may have only a vague idea that it is treatment to the feet for a therapeutic benefit. For the student training to a professional level a more detailed description and definition is needed. Because of its chequered history, reflexology is practised today in many varieties and forms and each of these may define itself slightly differently. Yet there are distinctive common features to all these varieties and the information which follows is an attempt to describe and define these.

What exactly is reflexology?

This question is one that you will often be asked by members of the public when you tell them that you are a reflexologist or by many of your clients when they first come for treatment. You will want to answer this question clearly when you give introductory talks on reflexology too.

Reflexology is a form of natural, holistic therapy based on the discovery that there are points on the feet and hands which correspond to organs, systems and structures within the entire body. This corresponding relationship is called a 'reflex'. A reflex is when a stimulation at one point brings about a response in another point or area. In reflexology, by using special pressure techniques to stimulate the points on the feet and hands, imbalances in the tissues, organs and systems of the body can be both detected and effectively treated to restore balance and well-being.

From this description, we can bring out certain important features about reflexology:

Reflexology is a natural, holistic therapy
As a natural therapy reflexology uses only the techniques of human therapeutic touch and interaction to bring about its results. It seeks to work with the body's natural, or innate, healing efforts.

As a holistic therapy reflexology shares an approach to health and the healing of disease common to other complementary disciplines such as homeopathy, naturopathy, herbal medicine, acupuncture. This approach, discussed fully in Chapter 1, basically takes a comprehensive and energetic viewpoint, one that sees that the person and their disease cannot be divided up into separately treatable parts, but must be understood and treated as a whole – mind, emotions, body and even spirit, each interacting and influencing the other.

Reflexology does not diagnose diseases nor attempt to treat or cure specific medical conditions
This statement may at first seem surprising, since we have above claimed reflexology to have a beneficial effect on health. However there is an important point of distinction here between the sphere of the licensed

medical physician and that of the reflexologist. Reflexologists are not trained to be able to diagnose and treat a particular disease or syndrome, such as cancer, TB, or heart disease; this is the duty of the physician trained in medical science and diagnosis. We are training to be holistic practitioners, to assess imbalances in the person as a whole and to treat by attempting to help the person's own healing energy resolve these imbalances.

Reflexology is based on the body's reflex relationships
Physiological reflexes

The existence of reflex relationships is well established in medical science in the physiology of the human body. There are several forms of these reflexes in the body, mediated primarily through the nervous system. These include:

- the simple reflex arc of nerve stimulation: for example, when an area of skin senses too much heat, the sensation is conveyed to the spinal cord via the sensory nerves and the motor nerves initiate a motor response of withdrawing the body from the heat
- the psychologically conditioned reflex response described by Pavlov: the behaviour of a person can become habituated or conditioned to responding in a particular way to a particular stimulus
- the reflex relationship between the internal organs and skin via the dermatomes and segments of the spinal nerves

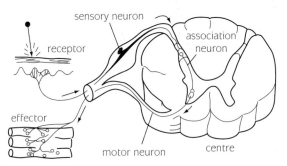

Receptor: responds to change in internal or external environment, e.g. heat, injury, pressure. Sends impulse through sensory neuron.

Sensory neuron: passes impulse from receptor to central nervous system, e.g. spinal cord.

Centre: a region in the central nervous system where an incoming sensory impulse generates a motor response/outgoing impulse. In the centre the impulse may be inhibited, transmitted or re-routed. The association neuron in some centres leads to a muscle or gland.

Motor neuron: transmits the impulse generated by a sensory or association neuron to the organ of the body that will respond.

Effector: the organ of the body, i.e. a muscle or gland, that responds to motor impulse stimulation. This response is called a REFLEX.

Fig. I.1 *(a) A generalised reflex arc*

- the reflex relationship involved in proprioception: pressure to the skin and muscles in the course of movement gives the body information about its position and balance in space and its response is to constantly adjust its position and balance. In addition, stretch receptors in the muscles tell the brain when a muscle is over-stretched and it responds by activating an inhibiting response.

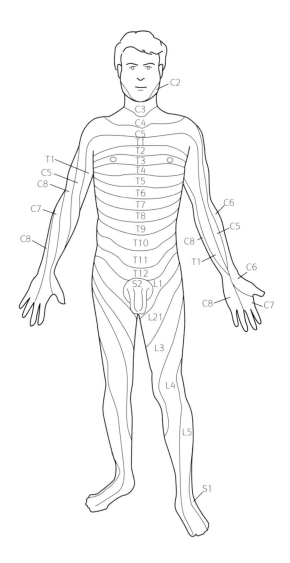

Fig. I.1 *(b) Dermatomes, showing the relationship of areas of skin to spinal nerves*

Subtle energetic relationships

Reflexology recognises that there are correspondences between points on the feet and hands and in the organs, system, and structures in the body as a whole. These links, or 'reflexes', are not visible or verifiable in anatomy and physiology nor by scientific equipment – as yet developed. But we know the effectiveness of these relationships because in practical empirical experience over many decades thousands of users of reflexology have observed the effects. Starting with Dr William Fitzgerald who identified longitudinal zone lines of energy in the body through which responses to stimuli could be evoked and continuing with the work of Eunice Ingham and others, we have learned that working certain reflexes has a beneficial healing effect on the corresponding organs. Such energetic reflexes cannot yet be 'seen' or measured, but they definitely exist because contacting them gets results.

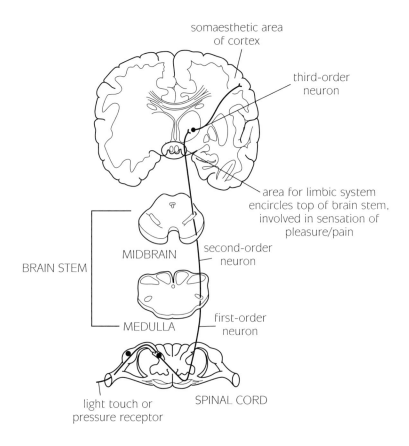

Fig. I.1 *(c) Sensory pathway for light touch and pressure*

How reflexology works

Reflexology activates definite physical and psychological responses
Physical responses

- Reflexology induces a state of deep relaxation and since it has been estimated that about 75% of disease is stress related, this is a major contribution to the return of health. As treatments continue over time this state of relaxation becomes deeper and more established.

- Reflexology stimulates a freer flow of blood and lymph supply to cells and tissues. This circulatory effect may not seem like much, but in fact it is crucial to health. Good circulation is of utmost importance in nourishing cells and eliminating waste from the body. The 'cleansing' and 'nourishing' effects of a reflexology treatment are a major part of its effectiveness.

- Improved circulation can be measured in terms of heat: after treatment a significant beneficial rise in temperature occurs which can last for several hours. The circulation of the entire body is thus enhanced.

- Reflexology stimulates nerve supply and the flow of nerve energy in the body, enhancing energy and vitality. This is entirely beneficial stimulation; one cannot over-stimulate the body through reflexology professionally applied.

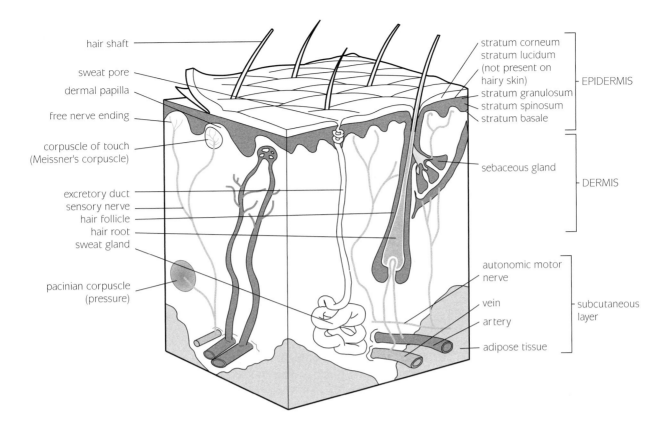

hair shaft
sweat pore
dermal papilla
free nerve ending
corpuscle of touch
(Meissner's corpuscle)
excretory duct
sensory nerve
hair follicle
hair root
sweat gland
pacinian corpuscle
(pressure)

stratum corneum
stratum lucidum
(not present on
hairy skin)
stratum granulosum
stratum spinosum
stratum basale
EPIDERMIS

sebaceous gland
DERMIS

autonomic motor
nerve
vein
artery
adipose tissue
subcutaneous
layer

Fig. I.2 *Sectional view of skin*

Effects of Parasympathetic Activity

Deep relaxation aids the parasympathetic nervous system in its job of balancing the activity of the sympathetic system, and helps the body recover from stress. Parasympathetic activity allows the body time for rest and repair and prompts many vital functions. When the parasympathetic system is dominant the following organ functions are improved:

1   The digestive system functions optimally, and hence energy is absorbed by the body.
2   The vessels to the heart are dilated, hence this muscle receives optimum blood supply,
3   Bile production from the liver is increased, improving digestion and elimination.
4   Motility and tone of the smooth muscles of the stomach and intestines are increased; passage of food and waste through the digestive tract is improved.
5   Secretion of enzymes of the pancreas and insulin release.

There are several thousand nerve endings on the feet and hands. Next to the lips these represent the greatest amount of tactile sensation conveyed via the spinal cord to the somaesthetic area of the brain's cortex. Touch stimulation of these endings increases nerve stimulation and integrates and enlivens the body as a whole.

Psychological responses

- Reflexology enhances the receiver's sense of well-being. Giving reflexology conveys a sense of unconditional caring. Touch is perhaps the primary medium of communication of love and esteem. Feeling cared for, a person responds with an enhanced sense of security and self-esteem which allows them to grow and develop healthily, to be healthy, to engage in loving relationships.
- Psychological health is improved through the sense of deep relaxation and enhanced energy brought by reflexology.

Reflexology uses human therapeutic touch

Reflexology technique involves touch given to points on the feet and hands by one human being to another and this helps give an extra, powerful dimension to the effects. In many scientific experiments it has been demonstrated that human to human touch is necessary to human health and well-being. (This topic has been covered thoroughly in the book *Touching*, by Ashley Montague.)

Reflexology as energy medicine

An interesting development is the growing evidence that the effects experienced by practitioners and receivers of reflexology and other complementary therapies may be explained by 'energy medicine'. Energy medicine focuses on physiology from the point of view of physics, taking our understanding a step beyond bio-chemistry to see the body as a field of energy. Physics explains that humans have biomagnetic fields surrounding them created by movement of electricity within the body. A magnetic field affects the spin state of nearby electrons, improves oxygen delivery to tissues and beneficially affects circulation. Studies have indicated that in certain conditions one person's biomagnetic energy may affect therapeutically the functioning of another's body by sending extremely low frequency pulses of electromagnetic energy through tissues via the body's living matrix, our webwork of fibres, filaments and tubes. This living matrix is a vibrational, dynamic network that covers all the body's systems (circulation, nervous, etc.) *and* is present in the cytoskeleton of each cell. By touching the skin, the therapist contacts the matrix and the pulses are transmitted throughout the body, because the matrix is a semi-conducting, electronic communication network. The body responds by improving its order and integrity and regulating its processes. This effect is what Eunice Ingham referred to when she said that reflexology helps the body to 'normalise'.

For further information, see *Energy Medicine: The Scientific Basis* by James L. Oschman (pages 42–55, 73–81) and 'Medicine for the New Millennium' by Roger Coghill in *International Journal of Alternative and Complementary Medicine*, Dec. 1998 (pages 19–20).

Reflexology detects and treats specific imbalances

As the reflexologist gives treatment to the feet or hands, she discovers imbalances in the reflexes. These may be experienced by the client as sensitive, tender or even acutely painful at the moment when pressure is applied. Or there may be no tender sensation at a reflex, yet the therapist can sense changes in the tissues that also indicate imbalance: tension, or congestion of tissue, or a grittiness – sometimes referred to as crystals, or changes of temperature which the client is not even aware of. Such tender, tense or congested reflexes indicate that the area of the body

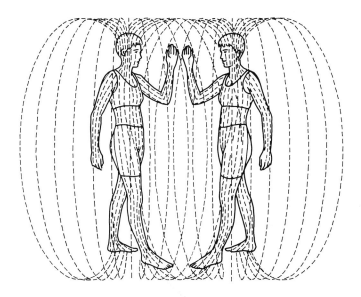

Fig. I.3 *(a) Biomagnetic field interactions between nearby individuals*

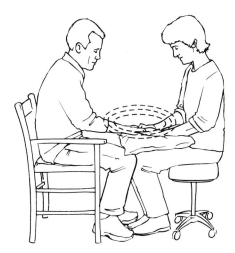

Fig. I.3 *(b) Biomagnetic field interactions in reflexology*

corresponding to that reflex is itself imbalanced. Such imbalance may be so subtle, or preliminary, that the client has not yet experienced any clear symptoms of disease. Or it may confirm the existence of a long standing imbalance that has manifested as symptoms of disease. By treating such specific reflexes, reflexology can both help prevent a more serious imbalance manifesting as disease, and treat an existing imbalance, restoring health and harmony both to that specific body part and to the body as a whole.

Reflexology promotes homeostasis and aids the Stress Response

Homeostasis is the body's condition of relative stability, i.e. its balance within its internal environment. Any disturbance in this balance is to some degree a type of stress and the body responds by adjusting its internal processes to meet the challenge. All these changes happen automatically and we are often not even aware of them. If there is stress of a more significant order, the body automatically adapts to the stressful situation. This is discussed fully in Chapter 1. After meeting the stress the body always seeks to eventually return to this state of homeostasis, the state of balance which enhances the life of its cells.

Reflexology, professionally applied, aims to return the body to this normal state of homeostasis, its internal harmony and balance. The body accomplishes its goals with the help and support of reflexology, through its effects on the nervous and hormonal pathways which together keep the body in balance.

Reflexology helps integrate our mind, body and emotions

Reflexology helps reconnect and restore the balance between our mind, body and emotions and to maintain those connections at optimal levels. Negativity, it has been said, accumulates in the most unused and asleep parts of the body where consciousness does not reach. Working on the feet with clarity and calmness of mind, a reflexologist can help a client relate the sensations to her present condition to the experiences, feelings and mental attitudes that may be contributing to the imbalance. The client begins to take responsibility for her health. Reflexology is thus a creative activity and a form of *re-creation*.

We can begin to appreciate what a tremendous place reflexology can have in health care. It helps to improve many conditions and also helps the body to function at its optimal levels, to recover and maintain its homeostasis, balance and harmony.

Summary of the effects of reflexology

- It induces a state of relaxation in which the parasympathetic system can function optimally.
- It counteracts the negative effects of stress responses on the organs and tissues of the body, allowing them to recuperate their function.
- It is a creative activity which helps the recipient get in touch with her own body's state of health and own emotional state so that realisations occur which enable her to alter her lifestyle so as to minimise the negative effects of stress and the challenges of life.
- It can be the vehicle for establishing a sense of being cared for and accepted, of being secure, that literally allows her to thrive as the vital being she is.

Only a placebo effect?

Sometimes the results of reflexology are dismissed as being due *solely* to the placebo effect, the implication being that the treatment itself does nothing, whereas medical procedures, drug treatment or surgery do, because their mechanisms are physically more observable and measurable, hence 'real'. Reflexologists need not be defensive on this issue because:

- it is now recognised that the placebo effect operates in biomedicine as it does in any therapeutic encounter. It is not just a subjective effect or psychological trick. About 30% of subjects given drug placebos in orthodox medical trials also improve within measurable parameters. Effects of orthodox drug medication and even surgery are also partly, sometimes even totally, due to this mechanism

♦ what is called the placebo effect merely verifies what holistic practitioners have long known – that the mind and emotions are intimately involved in any healing process, that they cannot be separated from the physical conditions of the body or physical interventions and that they can play either a positive or negative role. This has been called the 'biology of belief', i.e. that positive expectations, trust in one's attendants and a desire to be well are powerful aspects of healing. Norman Cousins, in *Anatomy of an Illness*, called it the 'chemistry of the will to live'. Two thousand years ago, the Roman philosopher Seneca noted that 'it is part of the cure to wish to be cured'. Today the intimacy of mind, body and emotions is being studied as part of the latest medical discipline of psycho-neuro-immunology.

A brief history of reflexology

Reflexology as we know it today evolved out of the work of Eunice Ingham, an American physiotherapist. Building on previous work by Dr William Fitzgerald and Dr Joe Riley in Zone Therapy during the early part of this century, she developed her unique pressure techniques and mapped out the now standard chart of reflexes in widespread use today. Her techniques involve stimulating certain points on the feet and hands in a certain way: the thumb or fingers alternate pressure with relaxation as they move carefully over every millimetre of skin in a smoothly flowing forward movement.

Before looking at her contribution, we need to also put it into a wider and historical context.

As Christine Issel has pointed out in *Reflexology, Art, Science and History*, reflexology is not the invention of any single person or culture. In fact some form of therapeutic treatment through touching the feet has been in existence in many cultures of the world from ancient times. It is because of this that Kevin and Barbara Kunz, leaders in the field of reflexology in the US, describe reflexology as a form of archetypal therapy found everywhere and to which no one culture can claim authorship.

Why are the feet so special?
Feet have been recognised as special by many cultures. Perhaps it is because they connect us so directly with Mother Earth as we walk upon her and draw from her powerful stabilising and nurturing energies. We know that we do receive electro-magnetic energy from the earth. Perhaps it is because the feet represent the opposite pole to our head and there is a polarity relationship between the two through the flow of positive and negative currents of energy.

In Jewish, Hindu and Buddhist spiritual traditions, the feet have been accorded a special significance. We recall the shoes are always removed when one enters a holy space and that Jesus chose to wash and anoint the feet of his disciples, demonstrating to them the humility and respect for all fellow beings he wanted them to emulate. We learn that the feet of the guru, the holy teacher and bringer of enlightenment, are held in most reverence by the disciple who humbles himself before them. Many paintings of the feet of the god Vishnu and of the Buddha testify to the holiness or spiritual significance attached to the feet.

It seems that the feet are at one and the same time the most humble and neglected part of the body when taken for granted, yet when rightly understood and respected can become the vehicles for great physical, even spiritual transformation.

On a more down-to-earth level, although we usually take them so much for granted, or are embarrassed by them, our feet do us a tremendous service. Bearing the entire weight of the body, they literally carry us through life.

Foot therapy in ancient times

According to Issel, the oldest evidence documenting a treatment given to the feet is from an Egyptian papyrus from 2500 BC with an illustration depicting medical practitioners giving hand and foot treatment to patients. Also from Egypt, from the tomb of a physician named Ankhmahor comes a wall hieroglyph depicting a form of foot treatment being given. Egypt was one of the most highly developed civilisations of the ancient world and made great contributions to medicine, sanitation, astronomy, engineering and administrative organisation.

We have as yet no direct evidence of it in Greek and Roman medicine but we do know there was a strong tradition of massage in these cultures, which may have included special techniques on the feet. A number of medical documents from ancient Greece, Egypt and the Near East may have been destroyed in one of the fires at the great library at Alexandria. After the Egyptian data, we have no firm evidence but might assume that techniques lived on in Europe through an oral tradition.

From Ayurvedic medicine, we know that the ancient Indians practised a form of pressure technique on the feet as part of their system of 'Marma' points. Similarly, Chinese acupuncture uses many points on the feet. We find the feet receiving special attention as a part of Indian and Chinese massage techniques. Native Americans too, for example the Cherokee tribe, have traditionally used the feet as a means of effecting healing on the body as a whole and have had specialised practitioners trained to do

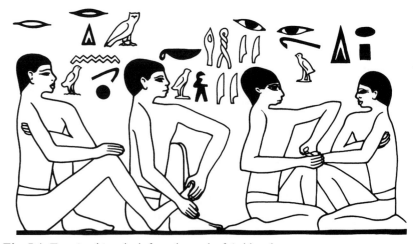

Fig. I.4 *Egyptian hieroglyph from the tomb of Ankhmahor*

this. Their skills have been passed down orally from generation to generation.

Early modern times

In Europe in 1582, a book appeared by Dr Adamus and Dr A'tatis on the subject of 'Zone Therapy'. Its existence shows that a form of reflex technique was known and practised, especially in the countries of central Europe.

Beginning in the early 1770s and gathering momentum since, health care and treatment began to change in western culture following the scientific and industrial revolutions. These fundamentally changed the way human beings looked at the world and their place in it. Drugs created in laboratories gradually replaced traditional treatments and a great optimism arose that all diseases – thanks to scientific discoveries in partnership with industrial and chemical technologies – would eventually be curable.

In a sense modern reflexology is very much part of this scientific revolution, for great advances in knowledge about how the nervous system works – including its reflex reactions to its internal and external environment – were made and are continuing to be made by medical investigators. A German physiologist was the first to use the word 'reflex' in his work published in 1771 on motor reactions in the body. In 1883 Marshal Hall, an English physiologist, coined the term 'reflex action' and described the difference between unconscious reflexes and volitional acts. In 1893 Sir Henry Head published his discoveries, made using patients who had traumatic lesions of the spinal cord, about the correspondences between spinal segments, skin sensitivity and internal organs: 'The bladder', he wrote, 'can be excited to action by stimulating the sole of the foot . . .'

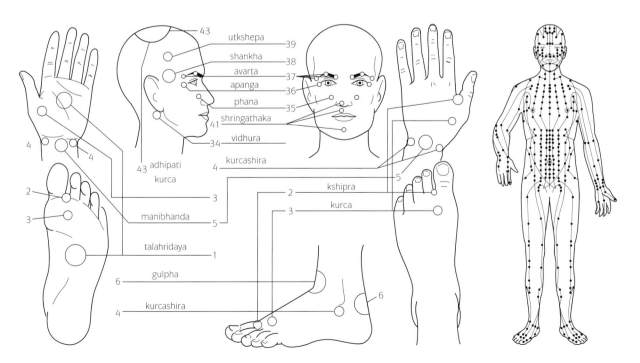

Fig. I.5 *(a) Some vital 'Marma' points on feet, hands and head, used in Ayurvedic medicine, (b) Meridians of Chinese acupuncture*

Two other British researchers, Charles Sherrington and Edgar Adrian, explored the way the nervous system co-ordinates and dominates body functions and activities. They shared a Nobel Prize for their discoveries. Adrian showed that the electrical intensity of the nerve impulse depends on the size of the nerve rather than upon the strength of the stimulus. Sherrington established that the brain and its nerves co-ordinate and control body functions through the transmission of impulses. He also developed the idea of proprioception. His book is titled *The Integrative Action of the Nervous System*.

Russia and Germany also made outstanding contributions to the understanding of reflex actions between body parts and developed various applications for treatment. In Germany research was undertaken into reflex correspondences. There these tended to be connected with the treatment of disease by massage. Around the turn of the century Germans developed 'reflex massage' in which the benefits of massage were credited to reflex actions. Dr Alfonse Cornelius discovered that when receiving massage, if the practitioner spent more time on the painful areas, the pain disappeared and health was improved. In 1902 he published a book, *Pressure Points, Their Origin and Significance*. In 1929 Elizabeth Dicke, a physiotherapist, developed Connective Tissue Massage, based on a concept of reflex zone massage, using the skin reflex segments identified by Head, called dermatomes, which correspond to internal organs via the spinal cord synapses. The existence of dermatomes explains how changes to the skin can be associated with disturbances of the internal organs.

The origins of modern reflexology
Zone therapy
Dr William Fitzgerald of New England is generally acknowledged as the 'father' of reflexology. It is believed he may have been influenced by the Native Americans of his region, for many tribes use foot pressure techniques for treatment. He may also have received some knowledge while studying in Vienna after his graduation from medical school in Boston. After his studies in Vienna, he worked at the London Hospital. Returning to the United States, he became head of the Nose and Throat Department at St Francis Hospital, Hartford, Connecticut.

While working with his patients, he discovered that when he applied pressure to certain bony prominences such as the joints of the fingers, or the mucosal margin inside the nose, he could produce a numbness in another part of the body. In other words the pressure had a reflex response. He wrote that he 'accidentally discovered that pressure with a cotton-tipped probe on the muco-cutaneous margin of the nose gave an anaesthetic result, as though cocaine solution had been applied'. He subsequently discovered many other areas on the tongue and nose which when pressed deadened sensation, and also that pressure to any bony prominence on the hands, feet or joints produced pain relief, and the condition causing the pain was also relieved. He went on further to discover that the parts of the body which had such a reflex relationship lay within certain longitudinal zones and that there were ten of these in the body. By applying pressure to points on these zone lines, he could create a reflex effect. He used various sorts of tools to apply sustained pressure, such as combs and bands. Fitzgerald mapped out these zone areas and called the science 'zone therapy'. He conceived that the body can be divided into ten longitudinal zones. Similarly to Henry Head, Fitzgerald found that working in a zone affected everything in that zone.

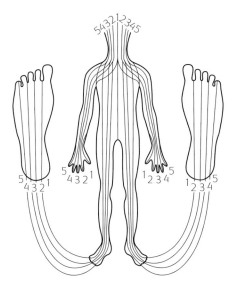

Fig. I.6 *Reflex zone lines of energy flow through the body*

Fitzgerald published his findings in medical journals and tried to interest his medical colleagues in his zones, although most of the medical establishment chose to ignore or ridicule his ideas. One physician who did not, however, was Dr Joe Riley of Washington, DC. He learned Zone Therapy from Fitzgerald and used the method extensively in his practice. He refined the method, began to locate points on the feet and the ears (similar to Chinese auricular acupuncture) and added four horizontal zones. Zone therapists employed probes, bands and other gadgets which Riley eliminated. Riley and his wife were interested in many areas of healing and opened a school in Washington teaching medicine, surgery, chiropractic and osteopathy, naturopathy, colour, and electro-magnetic therapy. They also lived part of the year in Florida where they employed a young physiotherapist Eunice Ingham, later Eunice Ingham Stopfel upon her marriage.

Eunice Ingham

It was Eunice Ingham who pioneered the use of reflex techniques on the feet and hands, gradually lessening the emphasis on Zone Therapy. Her unique idea was that instead of accessing the organs in the zone sections through other reflexes on the body's surface, she would use the feet. Gradually over time, through an empirical process of trial and error, she found that certain areas of the feet had a beneficial effect on certain organs and systems of the body. Thus she gradually mapped out these areas on the feet and hands. Interestingly, we now know that, second only to the lips, the feet along with the thumbs and fingers have the greatest sensitivity of any body part.

She called her techniques 'compression massage' and finally 'reflexology'. Trying many different methods to stimulate these reflexes, she eventually settled on one main technique, aided by several specialised ones. In this process she discovered that the particular diseased part would be stimulated to heal, instead of being numbed.

Eunice felt passionately that, if doctors would not be bothered to apply this technique, she should take her work to the public and non-medical

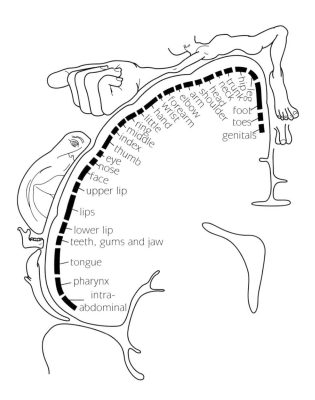

Fig. I.7 *Somato-sensory cortex showing degree of sensory stimulation to the brain from body parts. Note that hand/thumb and feet are second only to mouth/face.*

community, and she began teaching. She believed that people could help themselves to health. In addition to concentrating the techniques on the hands and feet, Ingham decided never to use any form of probe or other gadgets, as zone therapists did. Elizabeth Ann Riley, the wife of Dr Riley who supported Mrs Ingham's own work, also developed reflexology using a slightly different technique involving a rotary and twisting movement. In 1938 Eunice published her books, original works: *Stories the Feet can tell through Reflexology* and *Stories the Feet have told through Reflexology*. Some time later these two works were combined into one publication, which remains one of the most popular books on reflexology in the world today.

Throughout her working life, Ingham, and later some of her students such as Mildred Carter, were often harassed by the medical establishment and feared legal reprisals. Nevertheless, Eunice Ingham travelled across America many times between 1942 and 1974, teaching seminars and introducing the public to her self-help techniques. Even in 1968 she faced a court case in New York for 'practicing medicine without a license', but the charges were dropped. Two years later, aged 82, Ingham retired from lecturing and travelling.

Eunice Ingham died in 1974. Her work has been carried on by her nephew Dwight Byers, who, with his sister began travelling and teaching with Eunice Ingham as early as 1947. He has continued to publish her books, and has written his own book, *Better Health with Foot Reflexology*, first published in 1983 and now translated and published in nine languages. It is also one of the most popular books on reflexology today and is used as a basic textbook for classes and seminars throughout the world. Dwight Byers also established the International Institute of Reflexology, teaching the technique to professionals around the world.

INTERNATIONAL INSTITUTE OF REFLEXOLOGY
FOOT CHART
"Original Ingham Method"™

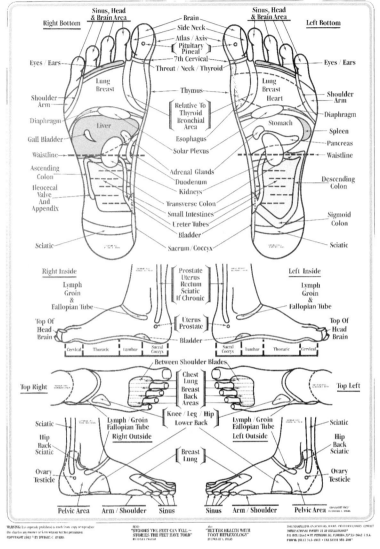

Fig. I.8 *(a) The IIR foot chart: map of reflexes on the feet by Eunice Ingham (Reproduced by kind permission of Dwight C Byers, President, The International Institute of Reflexology)*

Reflexology evolves

One interesting development of reflexology has come from the cross-fertilisation of western reflexology with Chinese medicine because of work in Taiwan and China by two Swiss missionaries, Sister Hedi Massagret and Father Josef Eugster. In 1982 the Rwo Shur Health Institute was founded to promote this integrated approach uniting the concepts of Chinese traditional medicine with Chinese pressure techniques applied to the feet according to Ingham's chart.

Another interesting variant of reflexology was developed by Robert St John: the Metamorphic Technique. This technique uses only the spinal reflexes and co-ordinates these to our earliest memories and influences

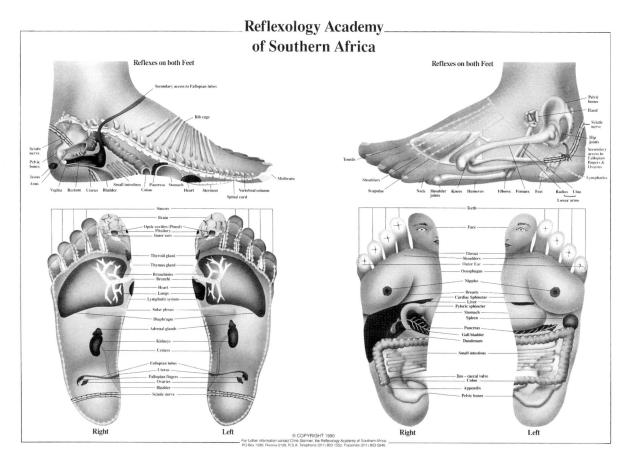

Fig. I.8 *(b) Map of reflexes devised by Chris Stormer (Reproduced by kind permission of the Reflexology Academy of Southern Africa)*

during the different stages of conception, gestation, and birth. These are seen to establish patterns which influence our development and growth during our lives, both emotional and psychological as well as physical. By working the spinal reflexes of the feet, we can release ourselves from negative patterns and thus heal.

In 1970 Hanne Marquardt, after training in the US with Eunice Ingham, brought foot reflexology to Germany, teaching its techniques only to physicians. She emphasised the transverse zones of the body: the head and chest, the abdominal and pelvic areas, demarcated by the diaphragm line, the waistline and the heel-ankle line. Reflexology is now a widely accepted form of treatment in Germany especially for disorders of the musculo-skeletal system, and functional disorders of the respiratory and genito-urinary system.

Reflexology was probably first brought to England by Doreen Bayly, when she returned from studying with Eunice Ingham. She founded the Bayly School of Reflexology. Anthony Porter also studied in America with Dwight Byers. With his sister, Anne Gillanders, Anthony taught the Ingham method in Britain and Europe for many years for the International Institute of Reflexology. He now concentrates on teaching advanced techniques (ART) to already qualified professionals while Anne has established her own school.

Reflexology today is popular with the public and respected by other health care professionals. The profession is working with UK government bodies to develop and implement National Occupational Standards for training in reflexology and to foster continuing professional development (CPD) among its practitioners. We are moving towards a model of integrated health care for the benefit of all.

ACTIVITY

Research the concept of integrated medicine from its inception to its present status. Discuss its advantages and disadvantages, promises and obstacles, with your fellow students.

Reflexology today

As we have seen, other ways of working reflexes of the feet have been developed in other cultures quite independently of Eunice Ingham's work. Today many practitioners continue to develop Ingham's original work, varying the techniques and developing new ones. Some reflexologists find that an extremely light touch is what works best, some prefer a circular type of movement and pressure, and still others have adapted the Polarity Therapy concept of linking energy points to working on the feet. Such developments are bound to continue in a field that is growing positively.

Reflexologists are also extending the areas in which this simple but incredibly powerful and effective hands-on technique can bring benefit. Some have begun to offer reflexology in such places as street drug rehabilitation clinics or hospices, others have taken its healing power even to war-torn areas.

Varieties of the reflexology chart

Since Eunice Ingham developed her chart, other reflexologists have found that other points may be co-ordinated to a particular organ or system and have added or even changed the position of some reflexes according to their empirical experience and new discoveries in anatomy and physiology. The two charts illustrated in this chapter are included to show that there is some variation in the exact location of some reflexes and also how they may be envisioned on the feet. One particular variation is that of the pituitary reflex, which many practitioners locate closer to the medial edge of the big toe rather than at its centre. Another variation is to emphasise that the reflexes also match certain acupuncture points on the meridians ending in the feet. For the student this may at first be confusing, but need not be. Let us remember that the charts are idealised representations of the links within a living organism, and there is bound to be some variation as practitioners work with living people. Let us keep an open mind and avoid being too rigid. The test is what works best or what works best for a particular client. The best approach now is for you to follow the methods and particular chart used by your course teacher and work with this for a good while until you become accomplished and gain a depth of experience. Then you will be in a position to judge which particular paradigm – or even paradigms – you wish to use.

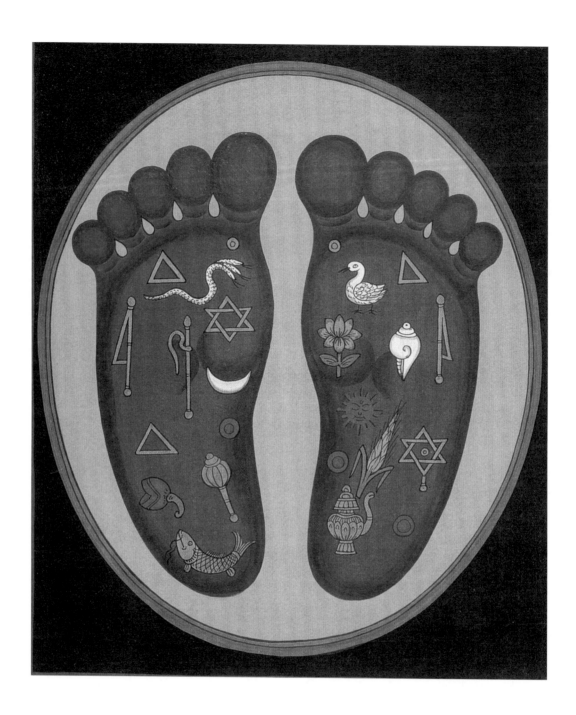

Fig. I.9 *Nepalese cloth painting showing some of the important Buddhist symbols that signify peace, harmony and the cycle of life and death*

Reflexology organisations

Building on the foundations of our pioneers, reflexologists have been getting together to foster the continuing growth and development of reflexology, ensuring it takes its rightful place among the recognised holistic professions which are becoming more accepted and integrated into national health care. In 1984 two British associations were formed, the Society of Reflexologists and the Association of Reflexologists. ITEC, the International Therapy Examination Council, also trains many reflexologists. These organisations act as professional bodies, accrediting training courses and representing the interests of professional reflexologists. Similar associations exist in Scotland, Ireland, and most of the member states of the European Union, reflexologists being especially well represented in Denmark. They seek to serve their members and the interests of reflexology as a whole by such activities as supervising the accreditation of training schools, offering continuing education for members, promoting research and publishing professional journals. For the public they publish explanatory leaflets, maintain a register of trained practitioners, and provide accurate information to the media, medical professions, and government bodies and other interested persons.

Reflexology organisations in the UK have joined to form the Reflexology Forum. The purposes of the Forum include developing co-operation and pooling expertise and experience among reflexologists for the benefit of the profession and the public. The Forum promotes research and encourages professional development of reflexologists. Over 80% of reflexologists in the UK are represented through the Forum.

At the time of writing, the Forum has been working on agreeing National Occupational Standards and a core curriculum for training, and has submitted its results to the Qualifications and Curriculum Authority (QCA). If accepted, these will be launched in late 2001. Training courses will become more standardised and be accredited and validated by appropriate professional and educational bodies. Ultimately the Forum intends to develop a national qualification for reflexology, and the individual bodies will consolidate into one overall organisation, rather as the British Medical Association represents all physicians.

In 1992 the European Reflexology Council was formed and two-yearly conferences are held. This has evolved into the Reflexology in Europe Network holding two-yearly conferences in member states. It seeks to influence the European Parliament toward official recognition of reflexology in these countries, to set guidelines for professional training, to exchange knowledge and experience, to promote research and to support reflexology organisations and schools. In North America, in 1989, the Council of North American Reflexologists was formed, holding annual conferences.

An American Reflexology Certification Board (ARCB) was established in 1990. ARCB is a voluntary, independent testing agency – not a representative body or accreditation board – offering national, non-governmental certification of the highest training standards. In the US, with no national health laws or licensing, reflexologists are regulated by the laws of the state in which they practise. Similarly, they are organised professionally at state level to regulate and promote the profession (to date twenty-four of the fifty states have such organisations).

The International Council of Reflexology began in 1990 and has members in twenty-two countries and six continents. Membership is inclusive and open to individual practitioners, as well as to associations and education bodies. Biennial conferences are held on a rotating basis among the member countries all over the world. The Council promotes

REMEMBER
MEMBERS OF THE REFLEXOLOGY FORUM: Association of Reflexologists, British Reflexology Association, British School of Reflex Zone Therapy, Centre for Advanced Reflexology, Federation of Precision Reflexologists, Guild of Complementary Practitioners, Holistic Association of Reflexologists, International Federation of Reflexologists, International Institute of Reflexology, Reflexologists Society, Reflexology Practitioners Association, Scottish Institute of Reflexology.

International Reflexology Week each September, facilitates the exchange of experience, art and practice, and fosters co-operation and mutual support among reflexologists worldwide.

Reflexology today is well placed to contribute a tremendous amount to the health care of our Earth's peoples as we move into the twenty-first century.

Further reading

The history of reflexology:

Issel, Christine. *Reflexology, Art, Science and History*. New Frontier Publishing, Sacramento, California. 1990.

Ingham, Eunice. *Stories the Feet Have Told* and *Stories the Feet Can Tell*. Ingham Publishing, Florida. 1992.

For scientific evidence relating to touch or complementary therapies:

Brennan, Barbara Ann. *Hands of Light*. Bantam Books, London. 1988.

Page, Christine. *Frontiers of Health*. C.W. Daniel, Saffron Walden. 2000.

Oschman, James L. *Energy Medicine: The Scientific Basis*. Churchill Livingstone, London. 2000.

Montague, Ashley. *Touching: The Human Significance of Skin*. Harper Collins, London. 1986.

Cousins, Norman. *Anatomy of an Illness As Perceived by the Patient*. Norton, New York. 1979.

Institute of Noetic Sciences with William Poole. *The Heart of Healing*. Turner Publishing, Atlanta. 1993.

PART ONE
THE FOUNDATIONS OF REFLEXOLOGY

Reflexology has its roots firmly in Western naturopathic tradition, the tradition of respecting and using the natural processes available to every human as the means of bringing the body back from a state of 'dis-ease' to a state of health.

At the same time, it continues to grow and to incorporate new knowledge to further refine its approach to health care. Its greatest asset is the high quality of its thousands of practitioners and their experiences with individual clients. Reflexology is a member of the wider family of complementary, holistic therapies which today are increasingly in demand by the general public and orthodox medical care systems. A well-conducted consultation enhances the treatment which follows. Consistent and accurate record keeping is important both for the practitioner and client, and also for the wider profession as a whole: it helps to build that critical mass of experience which validates the efficacy of reflexology. As a professional, the reflexologist understands that her approach to treatment is of great importance and that the treatment itself is part of the wider therapeutic encounter. The relationship between the giver and receiver in this encounter has important implications for the outcome of treatment.

REFLEXOLOGY AND HOLISTIC MEDICINE

After working through this chapter you will be able to:

- understand the distinctive approach of holistic medicine to health and disease
- understand the holistic concept of stages of disease
- understand the mechanism of the stress response
- recognise the place of reflexology within holistic medicine and its relationship to other holistic therapies
- recognise the parameters of a holistic reflexology treatment and the role of the professional reflexologist in the healing process.

The term 'holistic', while generally unheard of ten or twenty years ago, is of very ancient origin. It comes from the Greek word *holos* meaning 'whole'.

At least as early as the fifth century BC, Hippocratic physicians realised that it is necessary to 'know what man is, by what causes he is made and . . . what man is in relation to foods and drinks, and to habits generally and what will be the effects of each on each individual . . . so the constitutions of these men differ' (from the treatise *On Ancient Medicine* in Hippocrates' *Works*). This ancient medicine also emphasised that health was a balance, *isonomia*, and harmony, *harmonia* among different aspects of the person. In such writings we find the origins and hallmarks of the holistic approach as it is understood today. Such concepts have never really died out – naturopaths, herbalists and others have continued the ancient traditions – but today they have been given renewed meaning. They denote a distinctive understanding and approach to health and disease, and consequently the therapies based on that understanding. This understanding addresses not just the symptom or the disease a person has but the whole of the patient's nature in its multi-dimensional aspects.

The holistic approach: treat the person not the disease

Holistic medicine recognises that a person is not just a physical entity or merely a 'living machine', nor can she be neatly divided into separate social, cultural, physical, mental and emotional aspects which can be studied and manipulated in isolation. On the contrary, it takes as its starting point the need to understand the person within whom the disease is manifesting and that person as a whole. Being holistic means taking account of a variety of factors when understanding a person's health or disease: for example, her emotions, mental attitudes, lifestyle, diet, physical predispositions, past experiences, relationships. The synergy of all these things and more makes up a whole greater than the sum of the individual parts.

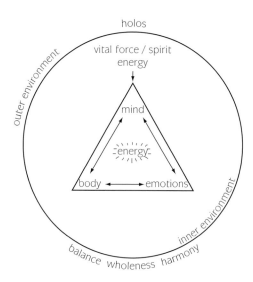

Fig. 1.1 *The flow of the vital force and the relationships of body, mind and spirit*

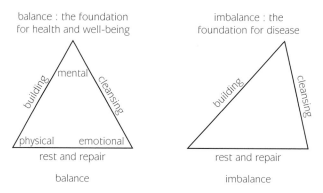

Fig. 1.2 *A comparison of balanced with imbalanced functions*

Disease as an imbalance of the whole organism

It follows that disease, even a short-term, minor ailment, doesn't just happen at the physical level, or to a single body part, for example, the throat. The psychological, emotional, mental and, some recognise, even spiritual aspects of the person are always involved in the disease process and likewise in the process of recovering well-being – the healing process. When any specific part of the body is diseased the whole body is recognised as being involved and affected, whether this is detectable at the physical level or not. This has important implications for treatment. While orthodox medicine may treat repeated tonsillitis with surgery or more often now, antibiotics, once the inflammation has gone, the problem is considered solved. However, from a holistic point of view the inflamed tonsils are in reality a signal that the entire body is in some way experiencing ill health and other aspects, in addition to the inflammation in the tonsils, must be addressed. When this is done, not only are the symptoms relieved, but the person as a whole becomes well, and returns to positive health.

Health: positive well-being or absence of disease?

A group of medical students was once asked to give a definition of health. The topic proved to be one they had not been asked to think much about before and sparked much debate. Finally the group agreed that concepts of health are based on measurements: certain factors are measured and if these come within certain established parameters of abnormality based on averages, then the person can be said to have a specific disease. So medical science measures us to see if we have disease. This approach does not necessarily take into account that the person may feel significantly unwell, yet have no measurable symptoms from a clinical point of view. If there are no measurable symptoms, then there is no disease present. Health and disease are thus defined exclusively in terms of quantitative measurements.

GOOD PRACTICE

When assessing a patient, seek to understand her particular symptoms within the larger, holistic context of her life and situation.

Holistic medicine takes a comprehensive view of the patient from the beginning and recognises that mind, body and spirit are all parts of one living being. It aims at a positive state of health and wellness, a harmonious balance among all these aspects, and not only the removal of disease symptoms, important though this certainly is. While recognising the value of all that medical science has achieved, it emphasises that the quality of the patient's experience of illness and wellness is of vital importance also and that the patient's state of mind actually has an important bearing on the physical symptoms. It does this because it has a fundamentally different philosophy about the nature of the human body and the causes of disease. Exclusively science-based medicine has recently become more interested in mind-body relationships in healing, which it calls psycho-neuro-immunology.

ACTIVITY

Start a health journal. Consider your own health: what are your typical illnesses or aches and pains, the things you are most prone to, if any? List these. Now think about what aspects of your life give you most cause for worry, strain or stress; these could be relatively straightforward things, such as the environment at the workplace because your desk is too low or high and causes back ache. They may be more complex: you've never completely got over a childhood shock. List any such aspects. If you feel one of these may be creating an upset of the natural energy balance within yourself put a star by it. Now think about little ways by which you might begin to balance yourself and who might help you in this. Note these down.

Progress Check

1   What is the origin of the term holistic?
2   What is one important distinction between holistic medicine and conventional medicine?
3   In what ways does holistic medicine offer a multi-dimensional approach to health care?

Fundamentals of holistic medicine

The vital force

Holistic medicine is first and foremost vitalistic. There is a life principle – a force or energy – within each of us that initiates and sustains our life, our existence. Its nature is ever to seek a state of health and positive well-being. In different cultures this principle or universal energy goes by different names. It is called *chi* in China, *prana* in India, while our Greek tradition called it sometimes *pneuma*, air, sometimes simply *phusis*, nature, from which we get our word 'physician', originally one who heals through the power of nature. The ancient motto was *vis medicatrix naturae* – only nature heals. In English this power is called the 'vital force'. In Chinese medicine *chi* is said to manifest as the twin energies of yin and yang. In Greek medicine the vital force moves the basic humours of bile and phlegm. In Indian Ayurvedic medicine *prana* manifests as three bodily humours: Vata, Pitta and Kapha.

This vital force exists at a subtle level and permeates the whole of creation with its life-giving energy, which is why we sense a relationship with other creatures and with the very elements of nature. Being subtle, the vital force is not always perceived directly by our five senses which are there to give us information about the physical world within and around us – hence it cannot be measured or quantified. But it does have an effect on our physical bodies. It is present within every living cell and makes life possible. It is rather like electricity: we cannot see electricity though it is always present about us but we can observe it with the right equipment and we can harness its power for our benefit.

The vital force manifests gradually from the subtle level, sometimes called our astral body or aura, to first the mental, then the emotional and finally the physical level, which is why these three levels affect each other so profoundly, and are so interrelated. Holistic medicine recognises this force and seeks to work with it. This is why we say that holistic medicine works with the mind, body, emotions and spirit.

Health: the dynamics of flow, harmony and balance

The nature of the vital force is to flow in a free and balanced way, energising every cell and tissue and the flow of blood, lymph and nerve energy. If this flow becomes congested, blocked, excessive or deficient in any one place – including at the subtle levels – this sets the stage for, or predisposes, disease to develop. Keeping our organism in an open, freely flowing state is keeping it in health.

Homeostasis

We recognise this natural balance at the physical level through the body's phenomenon of homeostasis: the body's condition of *relative* stability, i.e. balance, within its internal environment. This favourable internal environment, which the body strives to maintain, consists of:

- optimum concentration of gases, nutrients, ions and water
- optimal temperature
- optimal pressure in the fluid surrounding its cells.

Homeostasis is the physiological counterpart to the greater balance of all aspects of a person's life.

REMEMBER
Holistic medicine seeks to relieve symptoms of disease, but more than this: to understand and treat the individual as a whole and to return her to her highest state of health.

For health the different aspects of ourselves need to work together in a harmonious balance of activity. If any one aspect becomes either too excessive or too deficient, it gradually affects all the others and a negative imbalance is created. This gradually depletes the vitality of the body's energy, leaving it more susceptible to disease.

A process of renewal
Health is an ongoing process of renewal, not a fixed state of perfection. There is no such thing as perfect health nor should our goal be some impossible ideal of perfection. Our healthy state of well-being is constantly being challenged by different aspects of and experiences in our lives. The key to health is to understand ourselves, our particular balance of the different aspects involved, so we can order and live our lives, taking challenges in our stride without becoming too out of balance. Knowing ourselves, we enhance our strengths, while minimising our weaknesses, rather than living in ways that weaken us, block the flow or drain our innate energy, our vital force. Becoming more attuned to when our individual healthy balance becomes weakened and taking appropriate measures to restore balance before serious disease takes hold, we live to a greater potential of harmony, whatever our individual circumstances.

The body has its wisdom: the self-healing energy
The vital force is intelligent and so is the body through which it manifests. As it is, the principle of life naturally always strives for survival, health and well-being. Therefore, even though the body may give us symptoms of illness, such as headaches, fevers, and we call these 'dis ease' and wish to rid ourselves of them, these symptoms also represent the body's best method of dealing with an imbalanced state through its self-healing energy. Through manifesting such symptoms it is doing two things:

- first, trying to re-establish its equilibrium or homeostasis; given its present circumstances, creating the symptoms is the best – the most intelligent – means to do this
- secondly, signalling to us that there is a serious state of imbalance present which should be attended to.

Symptoms can now be understood positively as the body trying to grab our attention, to communicate that it is imbalanced in some way and needs attending to. We all know that feeling run-down is often the prelude to the onset of a really bad cold, fever or flu which literally makes us take to our beds – at last! We may blame it on a 'bug' but really we have been ignoring the state of the body, letting its vitality become low or depleted and it won't let us do this forever.

This is why it is not a good idea to suppress minor ailments with drug medications. This makes us feel a little better temporarily, but doesn't treat the imbalance that caused the ailment and in the longer term, weakens our health. Feeling symptom-free, we do not pause to adjust the way we are living that made us get ill in the first place. This allows the imbalance to continue, become worse or 'go underground', displaced to deeper tissues and systems. A long-term imbalance begins to drain the body's vital energy and immunity and fosters a state in which a more serious disease can occur. It is such repeated suppression of the body's healing efforts, such ignoring of the body's signals, that often sets the stage for chronic disease.

Understanding that symptoms are the body's best, most intelligent response to an imbalanced situation, holistic medicine seeks to restore balance and as a direct consequence the symptoms are no longer needed and are resolved. Holistic medicine seeks to listen to the body's signals and work with its vital, innate healing force in regaining balance.

The unity behind disease

Holistically, any disease, at its fundamental level, is perceived to result from a disharmony in the flow of the vital force – the flow is blocked, congested, hyperactive, or hypoactive. Disharmony in turn creates congestions or imbalanced activity in the physical body. Such disharmony becomes the context in which it becomes possible for disease to develop. The causes of disharmony can come from many areas of our lives: spiritual, mental, emotional, social or environmental, physical – sometimes a combination of two or more of these. We cannot always avoid these disruptions – life is meant to challenge us – but we can deal either positively or negatively with the situation, trying to re-establish our best balance. Whether the disease manifested is a cancer, a bout of infection or the result of an accident, we can seek to restore harmony.

Support and rebalance the body: the triad of treatment

This positive approach to maintaining health and resolving disease is one that may seem difficult at first but which brings long-term results. It supports the body in its natural activities of nourishing, cleansing and maintaining and in its healing efforts. It attends to the symptoms in a way that both relieves them *and* clears the underlying cause of the imbalances. These are the aims of reflexology.

GOOD PRACTICE

Fundamentally, treat the person not the disease or symptoms. Seek to restore flow, balance and harmony.

A basic approach is threefold:

1 energise the body to cleanse by activating the eliminative channels
2 bring about deep relaxation which allows it to unwind, feel secure, remove blockages and become open to positive change
3 tone and strengthen the body.

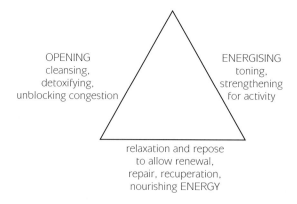

OPENING
cleansing,
detoxifying,
unblocking congestion

ENERGISING
toning,
strengthening
for activity

relaxation and repose
to allow renewal,
repair, recuperation,
nourishing ENERGY

Fig. 1.3 *The triad of treatment*

The role of the holistic practitioner

This holistic approach respects the patient as the most important part of the healing process. With treatments and advice based on holistic concepts, the patient learns which factors in her life may have laid the foundation for the disease and works with the practitioner to avoid these and establish habits of health and a frame of mind which enables well-being to return. Responsibility for healing rests ultimately with the patient. The practitioner's role is to support the body's own healing mechanisms and help create the right conditions for recovery.

ACTIVITY

Get in touch with your own vital force through breath awareness. For just five minutes, sit calmly in a quiet place and observe your own breath. Breath is the vehicle for the vital force. Just allow your mind to pay attention only to your breath as it flows smoothly and rhythmically in and out. If the mind wanders to other thoughts, as it will naturally want to do, just keep returning it to the breathing. Feel the breath as it enters your nostrils and consciously follow its path through the nasal passages, into the lungs and out again. Allow it gradually to become slower and deeper.

Now begin to relax a little more with each breath out, letting go of cares and tension. Feel that the out-breath is carrying these out of the body with it. Feel that the in-breath is bringing in life and energising you with its oxygen, recharging your batteries. Feel yourself balanced and calm, poised for activity.

Progress Check

1   What is meant by the term 'vital force'?
2   What are some possible consequences of the vital force being blocked or congested?
3   What is the significance of symptoms from a holistic point of view?
4   What is the approach of holistic medicine in treating symptoms?

Patterns of energetic balance: the constitutional, geno- to bio-types

Ancient Greek physicians taught that it is crucial to understand the humour, or temperament type, of each patient – his or her particular constitution of characteristics, physical, mental and emotional. They called it the patient's 'nature' (*phusis*). The remnants of this wisdom are still found in the works of Shakespeare and even in our language today. We may describe someone as phlegmatic or as having a 'sunny disposition'.

Our nature comes from our particular mix of some common elements, or basic components. The elements can be thought of as stages of matter from more solid, or Earth, to most rare, Air and ether. In ancient times, even the mind was considered a special form of matter. As in physics, what seems solid or material is really a question of the vibration of energy and each stage of matter is known by the particular quality of its vibrations. In each of us these appear in unique combinations, or patterns. We find this same concept in many medical systems – Chinese medicine, Native American medicine, Indian medicine, Western scientific medicine and in modern psychology (see the boxes below). This knowledge is even part of our everyday perceptions: the quality of fire is heat and we all recognise some people as being 'warm-natured', others as 'cold-natured' or having a 'cool head'; others might be typically volatile or 'scattered'. We are describing a truth about them which is qualitative, which describes the quality of their energy.

Psychology, particularly the work of Myers and Briggs, has identified personality types. Some of these are prone to certain diseases. For example the Type A is a workaholic overdoer who is prone to heart disease, hypertension or ulcers.

Medicine identifies three types:

- endomorphic – predominance of soft round physique, predisposition to digestive and metabolic dominance
- mesomorphic – predominance of muscle and bone, heavier physique, sluggish metabolic function
- ectomorphic – predominance of length, thinness and fragility with greater sensory sensitivity.

Chinese medicine recognises yin and yang types, yin being more introverted, modest and quiet, yang being more extroverted, assertive and passionate. Also, it recognises five patterns relating to the five 'phases' through which Qi flows in the body; each has its typical physical, mental and emotional characteristics and relates the human being to the wider environment. The phases are wood, fire, earth, water, metal.

The Bach Flower Remedies can also describe constitutional types if a mental state characterises the person's nature: vervain is typically the overstraining person, thriving on responsiblity; clematis is the rambling or daydreaming type; gentian is the perennially discouraged 'poor me' type.

Understanding such bio-types in a systematic way has much practical value in clinical work – as long as we remember not to use them as stereotypes but as means to understand patients more deeply. Each of us has proportionally more of a particular group of characteristics, thus giving the 'type', but we each have all of them to some extent and they all will manifest in response to the challenges life presents to us at different times. The benefit of such an understanding is that it enables us to live according to our higher natures, minimising any weakening or negative tendencies. As one client said, 'When you look in the mirror, you are seeing your own best friend and your own worst enemy.'

In a clinical situation, assessing a patient's constitutional type helps by:

- giving a structure within which to process all the information we gather about the patient in the therapeutic context
- helping explain why each person may react differently to the same set of circumstances, for example the degree of touch, helping our approach to be adapted accordingly
- guiding the planning of treatments and in judging the likely process an imbalance may go through as it returns to harmony. For example, a 'hot' person may have cleansing symptoms of a hotter nature (perhaps a mild infection or inflammation) than the one who is temperamentally 'colder'. It helps if we can anticipate this and advise our patients accordingly
- enhancing the therapist's self-awareness so we approach our clients with more clarity, knowing that our understanding of them is influenced by our own nature.

The table on page 13 uses the constitutional system of Ayurvedic medicine of India to assess the humours. In Ayurveda the energetic patterns are particularly well understood and defined. This table is a shortened form that allows you to begin to understand your own type or nature. Working through the table to discover your type provides a convenient and holistic way of exploring this whole concept. Having performed the assessment on yourself, you can use it to understand your clients better.

There are seven constitutional or bio types in ayurveda (called *prakriti*). These are derived from the characteristics of three biological humours or *dosas* in us:

- Air or Vata
- Fire or Pitta
- Water-Earth or Kapha.

These three humours can manifest as single or mixed types. In other words you may be predominantly a Water-Earth/Kapha type with only some characteristics of the Fire or Air types. Or you may be a mixed type, showing characteristics of mainly Air and Fire (Vata-Pitta) with only some Water-Earth ones. Some people are quite evenly balanced among all three.

Descriptions of the humours

Vata: the vital principle as movement, sensation; signified by Air and its characteristics.
A lighter physical frame (bones, flesh, thinner hair), colder body temperature (feels the cold), more dryness in body and in typical symptoms. A wind-like tendency to variation, irregularity, changeability, more sensitivity and reactivity. While lively and quick, Air types are more prone to worry, anxiety, fear. Air relates to autumn, to the hours around dawn and dusk. Symptoms are often worse at these times. Imbalances may show as loss of smooth movement or natural rhythm, such as insomnia, constipation, arthritis, muscle spasms and nervousness. Air/Vata imbalances are caused and/or aggravated by fear, isolation, cold, dryness, uncertainty, too much change (for example, travel).
Body system: nerves and senses, joints, voluntary and involuntary movements.

Pitta: the vital principle as energy of transformation, warmth and acute activity signified by the sun or Fire and its characteristics.

A medium frame, medium moistness, warm body temperature (dislikes heat), more colour, for example, red or blond colouring, skin blotches; a fire-like tendency to be active, sharp, penetrating; a fire-like assertive nature, competitive, thriving on challenges, ambitious, hard-working, practical and perceptive. While unsentimental, Fire/Pitta types are more prone to irritability and anger. Fire relates to spring-summer, to the hours around noon, afternoon and midnight; symptoms often appear or worsen at these times. Imbalances show as heat signs, fevers, infections, acidity, sharp pains, exhaustion from overwork, dependency on stimulants such as alcohol and caffeine.

Body system: metabolism (digestion, enzymatic activity), blood.

Kapha: the vital principle as nurture and growth, coherence, substance, grounding.

A stout, solid frame, with thick abundant hair, pale, moist, soft skin, cool to the touch; an Earth-like grounded and resilient nature, steady, prudent and thorough. While loyal and loving, Earth types are more sedentary, slower to take up new habits and ideas, to wake up in the morning, to digest food. Their tendency is toward attachments and to accumulation with strong feelings of grief or resistance to loss. Water-Earth/kapha relates to winter, to the morning and night time; imbalances often worsen at these times. Imbalances show as congestion, dampness (for example, phelgm), sluggishness, depression, swelling, cysts, tumours.

Body system: fluids, tissues

Each humour influences and interacts with the others as the vital energy flows into and through our bodies.

ACTIVITY

Using the table explore your constitutional type. Discuss each item with a partner, if possible, and be receptive to how others see you.

1. Place a tick by each characteristic that applies to you most, especially that to which you have had a tendency during most of your life, as opposed to just short term or recently. Then add up the number of ticks in each column to find how the humours are distributed within you.

2. Now ask yourself what kind of living habits, exercise, foods, music you can make use of to keep you at your best balance. For example, a Fire-Pitta type might avoid too much competitive sports which will only further aggravate the tendencies, and try activities that involve co-operation and team work instead.

 Progress Check

1. What is meant by the term constitutional or bio-type?
2. What are the three main qualities of Kapha and which aspects of physiology does it typify?
3. What recommendations (living habits, hobbies, foods) could you make for a Vata person that would help her to stay more balanced?

Humour assessment

	WATER (Earth and Water)	FIRE (Water and Fire)	AIR (Air and Ether)	
Structure (physique)	Large bones, chest. Tends to overweight.	Medium build and weight.	Slender. Small bones, chest. Light or underweight.	
Hair	Thick, abundant, often wavy. More body hair.	Oily, straight, blond, red. Tends to baldness as ages.	Fine, dark. Can be kinky (irregular).	
Skin	Moist, soft, fair to pale, thick, cool.	Moist, oily. Tends to moles, freckles, birth marks, acne.	Patchy, dry or rough, thin, dark, cold. Veins prominent as ages.	
Appetite	Moderate, steady. Prefers sweet-tasting foods.	Strong. Needs food to be content and to work.	Variable, but feels 'spacey' without food.	
Digestion	Sluggish. Food 'sits' in stomach.	Efficient, fast. Tends to acidity.	Irregular, worse with change or travel.	
Exercise and movement	Moves slowly or with reluctance, sedentary. Prefers slowness, conserves energy.	Active, prefers competitive sports.	Active but tends to restlessness or tossing, nervous movement.	
Stamina and energy	Strong. Slower to start but steady. Good endurance.	Moderate. Focuses energy. Tends to overwork.	Low or fluctuating. Quick to start and to stop. Intense energy, then fatigue.	
Stools	Moderately frequent, heavy with mucous. Tends to be sluggish.	Regular (one or more a day), large, soft, yellow-tinged.	Variable, affected by slight change (e.g. travel). Tends to dryness, hardness or constipation.	
Sweat	Moderate.	Easily provoked, profuse. Sensitive to heat.	Little, not easily provoked.	
Urine	Moderate. Tends to milky colour.	Profuse. Can be red or burning when imbalanced.	Scanty, less colour.	
Circulation and body temperature	Moderate to cool. Least sensitive to changes. Copes well with extremes (e.g. of heat and cold).	Strong, feels warm. Sensitive to heat.	Feels cold, and feels 'the cold.' Disturbed by uneven temperatures, changes, wind.	
Sleep	Sound. Enjoys long sleep. Slow to waken. Tends to excess.	Moderate, uninterrupted. Mind controls sleep, 'Night owl'.	Light. Easily disturbed, wakes easily. Morning is best time.	
Dreams	Romantic, emotional.	Colourful, involve conflict, passion.	Active. Involve movement e.g. flight, falling.	
Mental, emotional and life style	Thinks slowly, carefully. retains well. Good administrator. Compassionate, devoted, patient, calm, prudent, sentimental. Desires security (e.g. financial, love).	Sharp, penetrating, practical, articulate, knows own mind. Clarity of thought. Avid reader, likes to be busy, competitive, ambitious, judgemental. Teacher, leader.	Open mind. Alert, quick to learn and to forget; to grasp & to reject. Talkative, active, tends to be restless and overly sensitive, enjoys travel and change. Flexible. Communicator.	
Most likely negative emotion	Grief.	Anger.	Anxiety and fear.	
Areas of focus of imbalances	Respiratory, mucous. Congestion, inertia, water retention, weight gain.	Digestive, liver, skin. Fever, inflammations. Irritability.	Insomnia, stiffness, nervous or mental distress.	
Totals				

Reprinted from *Herbal Remedies* by Vicki Pitman. Chrysalis Books, London.

The disease process, the healing process

We understand that disease does not really manifest 'out of the blue' nor can it even be attributed solely to a pathogenic organism. In reality we do not simply catch flu from someone else. The pathogen is part of the cause but not the whole story. Perhaps our immune system has reached such a low state it cannot prevent the virus from taking hold. In this case we would need to examine and put right any imbalances in our lives that are lowering our immunity. We have many pathogens in our bodies all the time and our immune system usually destroys them before they take hold and provoke symptoms. But if this immunity becomes weak through a sudden shock or trauma, or we abuse our bodies for long enough and create conditions in which pathogens can thrive, then symptoms of disease can occur as the body deals with the situation. 'Creating conditions' can take place on the mental-emotional as well as the physical level of our being. Studies have shown, for example, that prolonged stress or depression can lower immunity. Stress from over-working can lead to exhaustion. Sometimes conditions are 'created' by factors outside our control. Emotional stress, such as from profound grief on the loss of a loved one, can be the trigger that finally tips the scales in an existing but long unnoticed imbalance – a disease is manifested.

Stages of disease

Naturopathy provides a very useful model for understanding the disease process. It recognises that there are acute, sub-acute, chronic and degenerative stages of disease, stages of dis-harmony.

Acute stage

This is a relatively superficial and minor stage. The body's basic immunity has not been able to deal with a pathogen or an imbalance so it mounts a more active defence which produces acute symptoms such as fever or inflammation (a local fever) with its accompanying pain and swelling. Such heat serves to kill many pathogenic organisms. In the process the body may create more phlegm or catarrh, or may produce sweating, or diarrhoea, depending on the nature of the pathogen or area of imbalance. We notice that at this stage such symptoms are usually located at the sites of elimination – the nasal and respiratory passages, the skin, the colon, sometimes the kidney-bladder, as in a case of cystitis. The body is in effect striving to eliminate the toxic matter through the nearest or most appropriate channel.

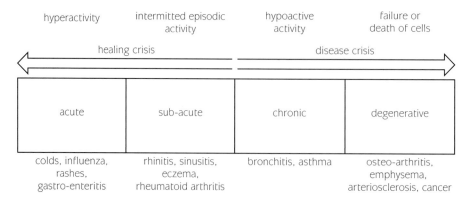

Fig. 1.4 *The stages of disease and healing*

If the body is successful and its self-healing reaction not suppressed, the body recovers and is in a healthier state. Often such acute, self-limiting illness appears when the body has become toxic to an excess, so much so that the normal channels of elimination – the respiratory passages, kidneys, colon, skin aided by the lymph – are not able to remove it in the normal course of activity. Such excess can be created by poor diet, or eating too much of the wrong types of food, by lack of exercise, or by a weakly functioning organ not able to perform its role.

Toxicity or congestion can also be created by an excess of negative thoughts and emotions. For example, constipation can be actually caused by a frame of mind that is obsessed with 'holding on' or with control. Long-term constipation allows fermentation to occur in the bowel, creating toxins that accumulate and eventually become the breeding ground for pathogens. This state can even weaken the bowel wall causing inflammation and pain or allowing the toxins to pass through and enter the bloodstream to be circulated to any part of the body which is weak enough to receive them.

If the body is not at first successful in ridding itself of toxicity or re-balancing itself, or if its efforts are suppressed, it may try again later to mount an acute eliminative process and we experience the 'disease' again. Such acute eliminative ailments are thus best seen as a healthy body re-balancing itself and treatments are aimed at supporting the body through this process. For example, in the case of reflexology, working the eliminative and immune reflexes to aid the body.

If the body is not strong enough to eliminate the pathogen, or the particular pathogen is too strong for a particular body, then a simple acute fever can become a life-threatening illness. We see this in the phenomenon that such diseases as measles, which is most often mild in Western countries, are life-threatening in areas where the overall health of the population is generally lower due to poverty and poor diet. Extreme inflammation can destroy tissues of vital organs and in this situation there is a call for stronger drug or medical intervention.

If the condition is not a life-threatening one but the body is still not successful, the body can be left weaker, with the imbalance or toxicity not resolved. It may pass to a deeper level in the body, or the body may encapsulate it in the form of a polyp or cysts, or localise it, for example in a joint. To this extent it has adjusted itself to the imbalanced situation and the disease passes to the sub-acute stage

Sub-acute stage
In this stage, symptoms may not manifest, or they may manifest only at a sub-clinical or low-grade level. The person can function well enough but may not feel really well. The body can carry on in this stage for a very long time. However, as there is either some congestion, excess or deficiency in some areas of the body's physiology, the effect of long-term imbalance is that major organs are gradually weakened as their functions become impaired. Acute eliminative activity may be localised in the area where the body has isolated the toxicity or where toxins have gathered because the tissues are weak; the body tries again to resolve the situation. There may be periodic local inflammation of the area, for example a joint, but it does not truly heal.

This stage is frequently what is picked up through a reflexology treatment. The patient reports no symptoms associated with a particular organ or system but the sensitivity or changes in tissues on the feet indicate that all is not well.

Chronic stage

In this stage of disease, weakness and toxicity have continued so long that major organ functions have become compromised. One eliminative organ often takes on some of the burden of activity of another weaker one, and can carry on for quite a while but eventually it becomes weaker itself through the stress of overwork. Thus the chronic stage shows that the imbalance in the body has become more complex and more organs and systems are involved. For example, if the blood is not properly cleansed through the action of the liver, plaque and atherosclerosis can accumulate in the walls of the arteries. This state can be in existence for a long time, unknown to the sufferer. All the while the heart muscle is gradually having to work harder to pump blood through arteries that are getting smaller and smaller. Reduced blood supply to the heart means it is not receiving the nutrition it needs. Gradually the heart muscle itself becomes weak and a chronic diseased state exists.

Degenerative stage

Tissues that do not receive the right amount of both nutrition and cleansing through proper blood and lymphatic circulation, or the right amount of nerve stimulation eventually degenerate. When organs and systems are in the chronic stage for long enough, such blood, nerve and lymph supply is bound to diminish and thus the tissues begin to degenerate to the point where the life of the organism is threatened. Locally such degeneration can occur causing loss of function, as in degenerative stages of arthritis. Such degeneration can be caused by cancer, for example, which prevents proper nutrition to healthy cells. If not reversed, death ensues.

The healing process and healing crisis

Many acute reactions, while uncomfortable even painful to experience, can be the sign of a healthy body throwing off its diseased state. Holistic medicine seeks to work with this process. It has often been called a healing crisis, crisis in this context indicating its original meaning: a turning point, the turning point from disease to health. We can also see it as a healing achievement and recognise that it means the body's healing, vital force is positive and strong enough to mount a successful healing process.

Stages of healing

Just as disease can be seen as a process involving many factors so too is the reverse: the return to wellness. In essence healing involves creating more positive energy in the body, and in the person as a whole. With this energy comes the ability to initiate and sustain a healing process. The place of reflexology is to help create the conditions which generate such positive energy.

Healing can also be understood as happening from the inside outwards. This is part of the 'Law of Cure' identified by the homeopath Herring. Herring's law states that healing occurs from inside to outside, from the top down, and in the reverse order.

> **REMEMBER**
> Symptoms at the acute and sub-acute level are the body's best effort to deal with imbalance, and its way of communicating to our consciousness that things are not in balance.

The first statement tells us that healing must come from within. There needs to be real inner change towards the positive in the person's emotional and mental state, as well as physically, for the healing process to begin. This doesn't have to be a dramatic, fully conscious act. Just deciding to come for reflexology treatments symbolises that the person is motivated and engaged in the process of getting well.

REMEMBER
Healing happens from the inside outwards.

The second statement tells us that the most important organs and systems need to return to healthy function first before healing can be effected in lesser organs and systems. For example, the brain, heart, liver then the lungs, or kidneys, finally the hands and feet, or more peripheral body parts.

The third statement explains that most recent symptoms will be the last to resolve and that previous unresolved imbalances, which have necessarily had to be contained without resolution, will reappear as they are restored to harmony.

Understanding this process, we will not be surprised if clients sometimes seem to get a little worse before they get better, or if they report the recurrence of a condition they had years before, or we see a skin condition that improves slowly at first and continues until the last traces disappear from the hands or feet. Our clients will be concerned about such apparent setbacks, but we will be able to reassure them that as long as the momentum of the life process is changing from negative to positive, such episodes are normal and part of the healing process. The symptoms may reappear, but this time they are on the way out as the body has the positive energy to eliminate their causes completely. The client may suffer again to a certain extent, but this time when the symptoms pass, she will feel better and more balanced.

Progress Check

1 What are the four stages of disease?
2 What is the purpose of the acute state?
3 What is going on during the sub-acute stage?
4 What does the term chronic denote?
5 How would you explain a healing crisis to your client?

Stress and the stages of disease

In his book, *Naturopathic Medicine*, Roger Newman-Turner draws attention to the fact that this understanding of the stages of the disease process corresponds closely to Hans Selye's stages of the Adaptative Stress Response. An endocrinologist, Selye pioneered research into the body's response to stress and explained his ideas to the general public in his book *The Stress of Life*. His work shows a profound awareness of the deeper issues involved in discussions of health and disease. Selye emphasised that it is our ability to cope with events and demands that matters, not the quality or intensity of these stressors; it's 'not what happens but how we take it'. He also distinguished between the 'eustress' or good kinds of stress that challenge us in positive ways, causing us to grow and develop, and 'distress' or negative kinds of stress that wear us down.

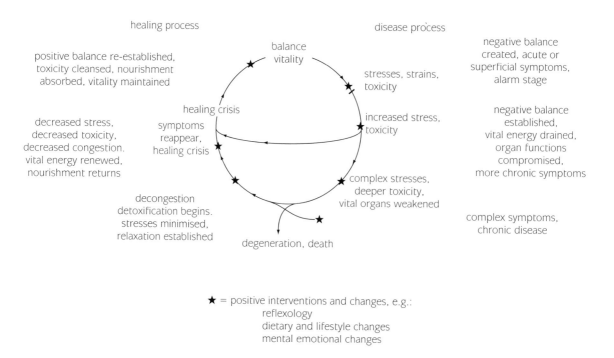

Fig. 1.5 *A flow chart of the disease process and the healing process, illustrating how positive changes can affect the course of the flow*

The stress response

Selye discovered that the body has certain unconscious mechanisms which are triggered when a dangerous or potentially harmful situation is perceived. This response is controlled by the nervous system and by the endocrine system. The sympathetic nerves initiate certain changes, and hormones – chemical substances secreted by glands to control and integrate metabolism and co-ordinate the response to certain stimuli – initiate others. Hormones are like nerves but their messages act more slowly and over a longer period of time. Nerves can be seen as the body's telephone system; hormones are its postal service. Together they govern the stress response. These responses happen in a certain sequence.

1 **An alarm phase** (corresponds to the acute stage): the body mounts its defences.
2 **A resistance stage** (corresponds to the sub-acute and chronic stage after a sustained period of imbalance): the body adjusts to a sustained situation and manages to cope and to survive.
3 **An exhaustion stage** (corresponds to the weakest level of chronic stage moving towards degeneration): major organ functions begin to fail, cells to die. If the resistance phase does not resolve the situation and return the body to homeostasis, a chronic stage ensues which gradually uses up body energy in maintaining an inherently imbalanced condition. Finally degeneration, ageing and death of cells or the entire organism.

Reflexology helps the body:

1   to be able to mount a successful stress response by enhancing the immune system
2   to restore homeostasis after the alarm and resistance phases. It aids the body's recovery from the negative effects of stress
3   to recover as much as possible from the exhaustion stage.

Things that may generate the stress response vary greatly. Even a seemingly small stressor – if frequently encountered and perceived to be threatening or even just worrying – may cause damage because the body is repeatedly being thrown into a stress response. Repeated smaller local stress responses can eventually develop into a general adaptation syndrome.

Stressors include such things as:

♦ loud noises: for example, constant telephone ringing, noise of machinery, tension of a production line
♦ threats (real or imagined): for example, job insecurity
♦ wounds or the potential for a wound: for example, a car accident just missed
♦ pathogens or poisons, including those released inside the body as a by-product of infection
♦ fear, or prolonged anxiety of any kind, any emotional upset.

REMEMBER
Repeated small, local stresses can develop into a general adaptation syndrome.

The stress of 'Life'

Selye discovered two important things about the stress response.

♦ It is non-specific – many different stressors can initiate the stress response and also, most importantly, the changes initiated by the stressor will affect the whole body. This is true of the responses by the body to any demand, whether caused by or resulting in either pleasant or unpleasant conditions. In other words there are innumerable stressors in life which can affect the body and initiate the stress response.
♦ It is a syndrome – not just one change but a sum of changes occurring, developing and accumulating through time. Thus accumulations of several episodes of stress or repeated stressful events can create a syndrome or group of changes. Selye called it the 'General Adaptation Syndrome'.

Effects of stress can occur both locally in specific areas and generally affecting the entire system. Local stress response is typified by the way the immune system responds to infection introduced by a cut or wound; we get swelling, heat, pain as the body sends in its defensive army to fight and contain the infection. We are here concerned more with the generalised effects of prolonged or repeated stress. A 'general adaptation response' is typified by what happens, for example, when we experience a sudden threat. The first stage has been called the 'fight or flight' response and is mediated through the sympathetic nervous system and the adrenal glands.

The mechanism of stress: the General Adaptation Syndrome

Stage one: alarm reaction, the sympathetic response

When threatened, your body prepares for fight or flight. The sympathetic nerves signal the adrenal glands to release hormones: adrenaline and corticosteroids. These enter the bloodstream which changes the body metabolism:

- blood is taken away from the periphery (skin) and sent to the large muscles and brain
- the heart beats faster, heart muscle contracts more frequently and more strongly
- perspiration (the cooling system) is activated
- the liver releases sugar into the blood to be the fuel for the muscles to stand and fight or flee. The body is in effect in a state of red alert
- the spleen contracts to make more blood available, red blood cell production and clotting ability increases
- digestive, urinary and reproductive activities are also inhibited.

All this is well and good; the body copes and responds and when the threat is over it returns to its homeostasis. The body has used the energy provided, the sugar is burned up with exertion, the muscles work, and the danger having been successfully met, the body returns to a recuperating state for repair and renewal of energy.

However, the problem for our health comes when this recuperation and restoration of homeostasis does not happen. We may encounter repeated stressful situations or not allow the body to recuperate adequately afterwards. It is important to remind ourselves here that stressors can be emotional and mental as well as physical. Our thoughts and emotions can initiate the alarm reaction. For example, we can be so anxious about our job security, or a sick loved one that our body responds with a stress adaptation. So how we perceive ourselves and the world around us is important.

Some symptoms of alarm reactions

Repeated alarm reactions can lead to many minor symptoms and ailments associated with the physiological changes initiated by the alarm response such as:

Churning stomach	Sweating
Nausea or even vomiting	Breathlessness
Racing heart or palpitations	Aching head
Trembling	Aching or stiff neck
Diarrhoea	Clenched jaw or fists
Dry mouth	Dizziness
Confused thoughts	Disturbed sleep

Although the immediate life-threatening nature of the stressor may have been met, the body still senses all is not well. At this point the stress response passes to the resistance stage.

Stage two: resistance

In this stage the response is initiated by regulating factors of the endocrine system. Hormones continue to circulate in the bloodstream. They allow the body to continue to fight the perceived stressor long after the effects of the alarm reaction have died down. In the resistance stage, the rate at which life processes occur is significantly raised – you could say that we are ageing faster – and although blood chemistry returns to normal, blood pressure and water retention remained raised. The continuing circulation of hormones in the resistance stage, if continued long term, puts a heavy demand on the body, especially the circulatory system and the adrenal glands. Adrenal cortisone is especially harmful; a high level in the blood is associated with diabetes, ulcers, and heart attacks and this hormone has been found to suppress the immune system, leaving the body's resistance to disease weaker. Many of us have the experience of feeling low on energy and then coming down with a cold or flu.

What is happening is that the body is now having to maintain a state of 'balanced imbalance'. In other words, it is not an ideal state but it is still the best response to the situation that faces the body – that of continued stress. As the balanced state is when energy is absorbed and used most efficiently, an imbalanced state causes an eventual draining of energy, undernourishment of cells and tissues and underfunctioning of organs. Such a state, unrelieved by adequate recuperation, eventually leads to symptoms of disease. These will manifest differently in different people, but they may all be to a significant extent related to chronic stress.

Symptoms and ailments associated with the resistance stage include:

Chest pains	Cold and flu
High blood pressure	Overeating
Abdominal pain	Loss of libido
Migraine	Phobias or obsessions
Insomnia, and/or tiredness	Depression
Wheezing	Accidents
Dermatitis or eczema	Alcoholism
Pre-menstrual tension	Excessive smoking
Loss of appetite	Low back pain
Indigestion	Persistent anxiety

Stage three: exhaustion

If the resistance stage continues long enough without let up, major organs become more and more weakened and their functions compromised. In the exhaustion stage, the internal environment around cells cannot be maintained, and cells begin to die. The adaptation has become chronic and finally degenerative.

The stress factor in disease and health

Having seen how repeated or sustained states of stress can so profoundly affect the body's internal organs and tissues, literally causing energy to be used up and the body's functions to work harder to maintain 'balanced imbalance', we can begin to understand why stress is now accepted as an important factor in many diseases. The resistance and exhaustion stages are in fact what we see in chronic diseases. Hence many diseases are not so much direct results of external agents, viruses or bacteria – or even internal auto-immune agents – so much as they are an indirect consequence of the body's eventual inability to continue to respond to challenges – stresses and strains of life – by adequate adaptive reactions. Selye came to realise that each of us has a reservoir of 'adaptive energy' and that this is depleted by chronic stress. In effect when this adaptative energy is drained or exhausted, chronic diseases result. Selye calls such chronic diseases the diseases of adaptation. They include such conditions as hypertension, diabetes, migraines, obesity.

Selye was careful to emphasise particularly that it is not so much the stressor agent that is important but our response to it. This is an extremely important point to remember. It means that rather than being passive victims of stress, of disease, we have the ability to minimise its effects on our bodies according to how we choose to live. We can protect, nurture and extend the life of our adaptative energy by the thoughts we entertain, by the way we respond to challenges, by emotions we enjoy, by the lifestyle we lead and by many other means. Many other thinkers have come to the same conclusions and they teach that it is not what happens to us in life that matters but how we respond to it, learn and grow through it.

This response also allows us to see that stress can be positive and is not necessarily always negative. For example, we need a certain amount of stress to grow and develop to our full potential. Exercise is a form of stress which strengthens our muscles and general health. When stress is – or is perceived to be – a form of challenge that encourages or prompts us to raise our level of performance, when it stimulates us or forces us to adopt new habits, it is a very positive thing. For example: working hard to complete a task, learning to speak up for ourselves in order to change a situation are other forms of positive stress. But if we perceive life events as stressful, or allow temporary acute stresses to become chronic and the dominating factor in our lives, we can allow stress to set the stage for many diseases. In some diseases, stress seems to be the most important factor, in others it is only a minor one but can markedly worsen the condition, or trigger bouts of acute phases in an otherwise stable situation. It has been said that stress is a factor in at least 75% of diseases. Thus learning methods of dealing with stress in our lives is one of the most health-enhancing things we can do. Rest, relaxation and recreation are the key factors in these methods.

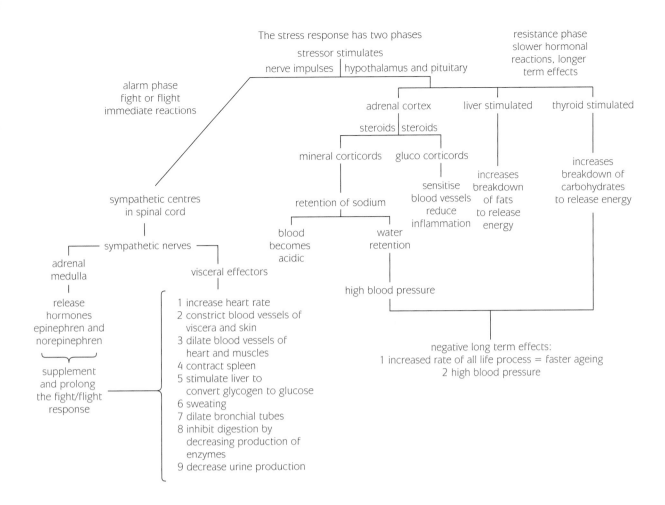

Fig. 1.6 *The processes of the stress response*

The basics of healing and health: nutrition, circulation, rest, cleansing, toning

From the description of the stages of disease and healing, we can also see that the key to the health of each and every cell and tissue of the body, as well as the body as a whole, is maintaining the body's own healthy processes.

Every cell, every tissue, every organ needs energy to do its work. Energy comes from nutrition, nutrition is carried to cells through the circulation of blood and lymph. Just as importantly cells, tissues and organs need cleansing, need to have the by-products of their metabolism, their waste, removed regularly and thoroughly, and this waste removed from the body as a whole. If not, it is as if we allow the waste from our kitchens and toilets to accumulate in our houses by not removing them regularly. Such a 'house' soon becomes a breeding ground for germs and disease, space is clogged up and activity is compromised.

For thorough cleansing the five elimination channels need to be active and healthy so that waste is excreted. These are: the lungs and respiratory system, the colon, the kidneys, the skin and the lymph tissues.

For optimum nutrition, in addition to high quality food, water and air, the digestive and respiratory systems need to be functioning well.

In addition, the healthy body needs both regular exercise and regular rest and relaxation. Exercise tones the muscles, increases circulation and elimination generally and maintains co-ordination of mind and body. Rest allows the body to repair itself, recover from stress and to relax the tensions which block the circulation and other body functions.

Balance creates harmony

There must be a good balance among all these activities, neither too much nor too little of any one of them: a good balance of mind, body and spirit, a good balance of outer and inner experience, of solitude and companionship, of work and play, of exertion and relaxation. By this balance and synergistic harmony we truly flourish and reach our potential.

ACTIVITY

In your health journal, reflect on one of your own diseases or ailments, whether minor or serious. Consider what factors in your life as a whole may have been involved in the experience for you. Having learned about your constitutional type, consider what aspects of your nature may have been imbalanced before the illness. What steps would you take today to bring yourself into balance as much as possible following the illness?

GOOD PRACTICE

Reflexology respects the person's whole being, body, mind and spirit.
- Its fundamental aim is to restore a positive, dynamic balance of these factors to bring about healing.
- It realises the patient's feelings and sensibilities are important factors in assessing the condition.
- By treating the feet and hands the reflexologist is treating the whole person.

 Progress Check

1 What are 'stressors'? Give four examples.
2 What are the three stages of the General Adaptation Syndrome or the stress response?
3 What effects do the continued circulation of hormones in the resistance stage have on the body?
4 How do the stages of disease and the stages of the stress response correspond?
5 How do the four stages of disease relate to the stages of the stress response?

Varieties of complementary therapy

Other complementary therapies work also with the innate healing energy of the vital force, though using different techniques. Each one has its own distinctive method and perspective. It is helpful for the reflexologist to be aware of some of these, either for herself or so that, when appropriate, she can refer a client for complementary treatment. Included here is a description of some of these therapies.

Herbal medicine: the use of plants prepared in various forms (tinctures, teas, decoctions, pills, capsules) to treat conditions of the body. The approach is holistic and the aim is to treat the whole person with the whole plant, often combinations or formulas of several herbs (not with an extracted 'active ingredient' as in drug therapy).

Homeopathy is based on the principle that 'like cures like' and uses very minute, diluted doses of herbs, animal and mineral substances to initiate the healing changes in the body.

Acupuncture and traditional Chinese medicine are based on the pattern of the flow of *chi* through the twelve meridians of the body. Through the use of needles through the skin on certain points along the meridians or using herbs and diet, the energy is returned to balance, and the organs and systems helped to heal.

Osteopathy and chiropractic believe that 'structure governs function'. They use sensitive touch manipulations, primarily of the spinal vertebrae, to re-align the spine and unblock nerve and energy flow from the central cord to the organs and systems of the body. Once this flow is restored general circulation is improved and healing can take place. Other specific manipulations may be used on joints. Osteopaths also use soft tissue work and often cranial-sacral techniques. The techniques are of particular use in back problems and injuries, or postural imbalances.

Massage uses special techniques of touch to the soft tissues of the body – muscles, ligaments, fascia and skin. This in turn affects the muscles, joints, nervous system and circulation of blood and lymph.

Shiatsu is a traditional Japanese therapy which, similarly to acupuncture, stimulates points along the meridian lines. Stimulation is given using a combination of pressure techniques using hands, elbows, knees and feet.

Aromatherapy uses the extracted volatile essences of aromatic plants to initiate healing. These essential oils are given using massage and other means such as inhalation, baths, and, rarely, ingestion.

Bach flower remedies are prepared from flowering trees, plants and shrubs and prescribed for their effects on the mood or mental state of the patient, which in turn is understood to cause a physical disease.

Nutritional therapy, understanding that diet is the basic foundation of health and profoundly affects the processes of growth, repair and energy, gives advice on the correct dietary needs according to individual requirements. These vary among people and also with age, lifestyle, size, weight and gender.

Psychotherapy, autogenics, counselling, NLP (Neuro-Linguistic Programming) and other similar therapies approach health primarily through the psychological-emotional-mental levels and aim to reconnect the clients with their own healing energy through a variety of techniques. For example, discussing problems or situations, guided dream imagery, relaxation and creative visualisation.

Yoga, T'ai chi and Qi gong are methods of physical exercises, postures (*asanas*) and movements, and related breathing techniques which aim to restore or maintain the balanced flow of *prana* or *chi* through the body. They can be used for general exercise or for specific therapeutic goals under the guidance of a qualified teacher.

Ayurveda, the traditional medical system of India, views the body in terms of three biological humours or *tri-dosas* which relate to the natural elements of the creation, to consciousness and to the vital force as *prana*. Using herbs, diet, bodywork, marma point stimulation, colour and other therapies, it prompts healing through a balancing of the person's *dosas*.

ACTIVITY

Research the availability of complementary therapies in your area. In addition to the ones above, look out for practitioners of crystal therapy, spiritual healing, colour therapy, applied kinesiology and any others. Write for leaflets or visit the clinics to find out the approach of the therapy, how much sessions cost and the typical problems the therapy can help.

Key Terms

You need to know what these words mean. Go back through the chapter or check in the glossary to find out.

- Holistic
- Vital force
- Stages of disease
- Elimination channels
- Adaptation
- Synergy
- Homeostasis
- Healing crisis/achievement
- Stress response

Further reading

Holistic paradigms of health:

Orthodox medicine: Pietroni, Patrick. *The Greening of Medicine*. Victor Gollancz, London. 1990.

Featherstone, Cornelia and Forsythe, Lori. *Medical Marriage: The New Partnership*. Findhorn Press, London. 1997.

Naturopathy:

Newman-Turner, Roger. *Naturopathic Medicine*. Thorsons/Harper Collins, London. 1990.

Herbal medicine:

Pitman, Vicki. *Herbal Remedies*. Chrysalis Books, London. 2002

Chinese medicine:

Kaptchuk, Ted. *The Web That Has No Weaver*, revised edition. Rider, London. 2000.

Ayurvedic medicine:

Lad, Vasant. *Ayurved: The Science of Self-Healing*. Lotus Press, Wilmot, WI. 1984.

Morrison, Judith. *The Book of Ayurveda*. Gaia Books, London. 1994.

There are many books on the stress response and relaxation techniques. Here are two classics and one that explores them in a specific disease context:

Selye, Hans. *The Stress of Life*. McGraw-Hill, London. 1990. (the seminal work in this field)

Benson, H. *The Relaxation Response*. Avon, London. 1976.

Ornish, Dean. *Dr Dean Ornish's Program for Reversing Heart Disease*. Ivy Books, New York. 1996.

2 THE NATURE OF THE THERAPEUTIC RELATIONSHIP

After working through this chapter you will be able to:

♦ understand the process of interaction between the holistic therapist and client
♦ understand the importance of developing self-awareness
♦ understand the importance of working from your centre of awareness
♦ understand the different responsibilities and boundaries existing between therapist and client.

While using a simple technique, reflexology involves many different factors. One of the most important of these is the relationship between the therapist and client – the therapeutic relationship. The nature of this relationship has significant implications for the healing process.

In addition to the practical treatment, the therapist brings to the process of healing something of their own energy, their own state of mind and being. The quality of this energy is significant. We need to be aware that when treating a patient or client (different people prefer one of these terms) we are entering a relationship with her and we want to make and keep this a positive one.

While we wish to relieve symptoms and restore health using the reflexology technique, our higher goal is to guide or support the patient to discover and/or understand her own nature better – her own state of balance, and further, what factors disrupt that balance and can lead ultimately to disease.

Energies in the therapeutic relationship

Holistically we recognise three energies present in a therapeutic relationship and these combine dynamically to foster healing and health:

♦ the energy of the client
♦ the energy of the practitioner, and underneath or behind these
♦ the energy of the healing power of the vital force itself.

REMEMBER
Any imbalance means the vital force of the person is to an extent flowing in a negative pattern - a pattern which eventually weakens the body's health and brings about its present state.

The client's energy
The client brings her own energy into this relationship. In the first instance, because she does not feel well, the client is to varying degrees vulnerable. Whether her energy appears low or hyperactive, distracted or congested, it is to a significant extent imbalanced and to that extent she needs our help and support. Understanding this pattern of energy flow will help us understand the likely imbalances and causes for these in each client. What we learn from treating the feet helps us further in this understanding.

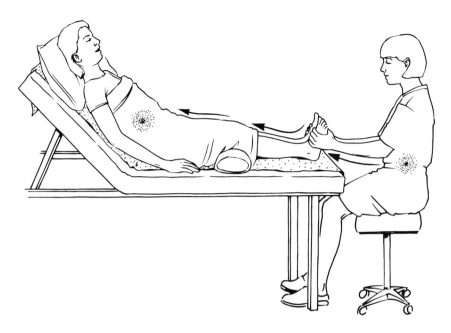

Fig. 2.1 *Energy flow in the therapeutic relationship*

Clients vary but all need to be part of the treatment

Among the clients who come to us, we will find that some may be already quite self-aware and just need a little support for their own growth and healing. Some may be very stuck and stagnant in the habits that have brought them to their present condition. Others have suffered a trauma which will take some time to resolve, and more prolonged treatment, deeper work may be required to change their pattern from a negative to a positive one. Some clients are very 'head oriented', want to participate actively in the process and respond best if given a lot of information along with treatment; they may bring a lot of information about themselves to treatment. Others respond best by just receiving the treatment and the deep relaxation that goes with it, without articulating what they feel. Still others, while initially enthusiastic, in practice may find it more difficult to commit to the necessary treatment or initiate changes that are indicated, beneficial though these may be in theory. They may tend to react quickly or strongly to the stimulation of the treatment.

Some clients, especially those with several different areas of concern, may not be aware of how much progress they have made. If we ask them how they feel, they may not indicate much progress. Yet if we ask them about some specific points, for example, changes in sleep pattern, or in frequency of occurrence of symptoms, and compare their reported sensations with those of their first consultation, we will be able to show them that considerable progress has been made. This is often important to make the client more open to the possibility of change and give the staying power and determination to see the healing process through to its conclusion.

All clients need at some level to engage in the processes of change that will lead to healing, to co-operate with the practitioner in a return to health. This enhances the effects of the treatment. As the treatments continue, clients and their circumstances change and the therapist will adapt the treatment and advice to new circumstances. But the therapist should not feel totally responsible for the progress or lack thereof by the client. A large part of this responsibility lies with the client.

Client in charge

Ultimately, the power for healing lies in the client's own hands. Sometimes a client may not like to recognise this and tend to look on the practitioner as the expert who will put things right or transfer all their hopes onto the practitioner, much as a child trusts in a parent. As holistic practitioners we recognise if this happens and can guide the client to a more adult role of responsibility and to knowledge of their own inner resources by responding as an adult from our place of centredness; we avoid unconsciously allowing ourselves to exploit the client's vulnerability for our own self-esteem, or accept any undue share of responsibility. It is not we who do the healing but the client and her own vital force. The therapist facilitates the client's power of self-healing.

Respecting the client's space

Being 'in charge' also means the client is free to initiate changes in her own time. Our job is not to impose rigid ideas on the client but to advise while she chooses what feels right for her to take on board at the time.

After we have done an initial assessment and formed our aims or strategy for treatment, we will discuss this treatment plan or pattern with the client, explaining how we propose to proceed, for example, how often we recommend treatment and for how long, and confirming if this is acceptable. This also allows the client to be part of the process.

> **REMEMBER**
> The responsibility of the client: co-operation and participation
> The power of the client: being in charge of her own health; having access to her own healing power
> The vulnerability of the client: needing our detached and loving care.

 Progress Check

1 How might it help the healing process if the client feels involved?
2 What does respecting the client involve?
3 How might we use knowledge of a client's energy pattern to help us know what to expect from her?

The therapist's energy

As the therapist acts as a catalyst for releasing the healing energy within the client, it is important for our input to be as positive as possible, and for this we need to develop self-awareness and the skill of working from a point of inward centredness.

Responding not reacting

Working from an inner point of balance or centredness means that no matter what type of client comes to us, or what the nature of their imbalances, we can respond positively. If we do not know ourselves well first, we may simply 'react' to or with the client. This means involving ourselves in that energy imbalance.

Working from our centre keeps us from losing our balance as we work and from having our own energy drained. Self-awareness is important, because if we are not clear in ourselves about who we are and where we are coming from – about our own issues, predispositions and habitual attitudes – we might unwittingly impose these on the client, or misunderstand what the client is trying to communicate to us. Being clear avoids this. Finally, it enhances the flow of healing energy.

Protecting our space

Self-awareness and being centred helps to protect us from merely absorbing any negative energy from the client. We are mindful not to take on the problems of the client, not to take them too much to heart, or to allow the client to transfer any negativity to us.

If we still find that we are tending to take concerns over our clients too much to heart, there are other means of creating a sense of detachment and separation. One of these is to ritualise the separation in some way. For example, we can make it a point that, as we wash our hands immediately after treatment, we consciously visualise that the water is cleansing the energy between us and the client.

GOOD PRACTICE

Take a few moments to do five deep relaxing breaths between clients. As you breathe in, repeat to yourself the word 'peace'. As you breathe out, say to yourself the word 'calm'.

The therapist's responsibility

To give treatments in this way means the therapist needs to take responsibility for her own health at the level of body, mind, spirit. 'Working' on ourselves can be done in many ways. Some practitioners prefer or need to have treatments from another therapist or counselling to identify and balance patterns of negativity. For some, practices such as meditation, yoga, t'ai chi, breathing techniques, relaxation, bio-feedback, or engaging in regular periods of inner reflection help to bring understanding about our own patterns and help us to access our own inner resources. Receiving treatments and practising 'on ourselves' helps develop self-awareness and inner strength and, as an integral part of the therapist's life, benefit ourselves and our clients.

For example, if we are going to be recommending our clients to relax more, we need to know and experience for ourselves what deep relaxation means. We need to be able to practise it as needed. To foster ideas of positive health in our clients we need to live them in our own lives. To lead clients to find their balance we need to have awareness of our own balance. Of course such goals involve a lifelong endeavour which needs constant renewal, but we can all make a start.

Self-awareness has very important practical effects. Only by working from a position of balance can we offer our skills in a loving but detached manner. From this position there is no question of either misusing the client's trust and vulnerability or transferring our own preoccupations to the client. For example, if we have just experienced a

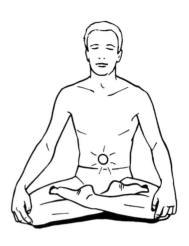

Fig. 2.2 *(a) Yoga meditation and breath awareness*

certain success with a particular treatment on ourselves – for example we may have relieved our headache by working on the liver reflex – we are naturally enthusiastic about it. If we are not careful we may automatically transfer our enthusiasm and use this technique on the next client presenting with a headache, without keeping an open mind and letting her feet and nature tell us where the origin of the problem lies in that individual. If we are conscious and work from our centre, we can avoid such unconscious transference.

The real world is not perfectly harmonious; we are all affected by what goes on in and around us. However, we can counter the tendency to let our world spill over to our clients. For example, even if we are having a bad day personally, we must still be present in a calm frame of mind for giving treatment. Or if not, knowing ourselves well enough to sense this is not possible, we can make arrangements to give treatments at another time.

Integrity and working within the limits of training

Integrity can mean many things, for example, to act for the client's best interest, not our own, and to maintain strict confidentiality. It can also mean respecting and acting honestly toward other therapists and other disciplines within the healing arts. It can mean working within the limits of our training, knowing when to refer to another practitioner. Inwardly, as we have seen, it means engaging in our own journey towards health and well-being on all levels. The word 'integrity' comes from a Latin word meaning wholeness, completeness, even purity. You could say having integrity means being so connected to our true selves that we naturally behave in a genuinely honest way.

Reflexology is a powerful tool for health and healing. However, this does not mean it is a cure-all for every condition. Promising to cure every condition would be a breach of trust between therapist and client. Knowing this, reflexologists work within certain guidelines.

♦ We never claim to 'cure' any disease or condition. Diagnosing and curing diseases is the province of the medical physician, not the reflexologist.

> **REMEMBER**
>
> As practitioners we too are moving toward our own wholeness, outwardly continuing to develop and improve our skills of touch and understanding, inwardly endeavouring to know ourselves, our own strengths and weaknesses, our potentials as well as our limitations.

- We must never advise clients to stop taking any medications. This should only be done through the patient's consultation with their doctor. However, we may contact the doctor, with the client's permission, and inform him or her about reflexology and its probable positive effects on the body.
- We must not give or advise on treatments for which we are not fully trained and qualified. For example, if we are not aromatherapists, we should not use aromatherapy in our practice.
- When we feel reflexology or our own expertise has come to a point where it is no longer a catalyst for change with a particular client, bearing the client's best interests in mind, we have the integrity to accept this and refer the client to some other form of treatment that we think will help.
- When we feel that understanding a condition or symptom is beyond our expertise or we suspect a serious medical condition that merits a doctor's examination, we do not hesitate to advise the client to check with their GP.

GOOD PRACTICE

Recognise the limits of your training and be prepared to refer clients to a doctor or other practitioner when necessary.

Working within the limits of training also means that as your experience and competence grow and develop, as you undertake to regularly up-date and extend your skills, as you help more and more clients, your expertise and limits of training naturally expand. You may responsibly treat after five years someone that you may not have considered it appropriate to treat in your early years of practice.

REMEMBER

The responsibility of the practitioner: skills confidence, self-awareness
The power of the practitioner: expertise, access to inner resources
The vulnerability of the practitioner: needing support from others and protection from within.

ACTIVITY

With a fellow student or students, identify and discuss five conditions or situations in which you would refer a client to another practitioner or medical doctor.

Progress Check

1. Why is it important not to diagnose disease conditions or claim to cure them with reflexology?
2. What are five possible circumstances in which you would consider referring a client to another type of alternative medicine practitioner?
3. Why is it important not to advise a client to reduce any medication prescribed by their GP?
4. When might you advise a client to have a check-up from their GP?

The healing energy of the vital force

The third energy in the therapeutic relationship is that of the vital force itself. Through our skills of reflexology we try to release any blockages to this energy and promote its free flow. We try to bring our clients in touch with this inner resource. This is the true healing power in the client.

A good motto is 'expect the unexpected'. It is our duty to be well trained and capable, but let us remember that there are many factors operating in our clients' lives and changes can come from any one of these. Exactly why the positive energy begins to flow strongly and the healing begins is sometimes a mystery. Our job is to create the conditions in which it is at least possible for the creative process of change and renewal to flow.

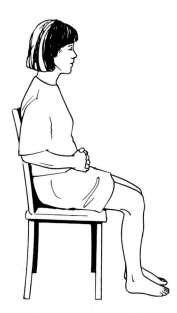

Fig. 2.2 *(b) Relaxation through breath awareness while seated and breathing into the solar plexus*

ACTIVITY
Practise this centring exercise.

1   Place your hand on your abdomen just below the navel. Breathe five times into your lower abdomen, feeling that with each breath out you are releasing all the tension in your body, all discomfort, all this is flowing out with the out-breath. With the in-breath, you are renewing your energy; feel the breath as it comes in through your nostrils and down into the deep lungs to your centre around the navel. From there it diffuses to every cell of your body, carrying oxygen and the energy of the vital force. Each in-breath renews the body with fresh oxygen and vitality. Each in-breath flows into your nostrils, down into your lungs to your navel area and from there, diffuses throughout the body. Every organ, tissue and cell is revitalised and nourished with this healing breath. Through this conscious breathing you can even increase the reservoir of energy within yourself.

2 After five breaths, rest a few moments in normal breathing, absorbing the feeling of relaxation and calm. Feel yourself connected to your inner core, a place of strength and calm, a place not of 'doing' but 'being'. This is your centre of gravity, your centre of balance and poise; the fulcrum of your activity.

3 Continue to breathe calmly into your centre, feeling warm, heavy, relaxed. Be aware also that you feel renewed, vital and poised for whatever may come to you.

Now that you have found this place of dynamic poise, know that you can return to it whenever you need - by using your breath and your awareness. Whenever you want to, using your breath, you can calm your mind and emotions and recharge your energy by returning to your centre of calmness, peace and strength. The more you practise this, the easier it becomes to access your inner strength and power, which is always there for you whenever you need it.

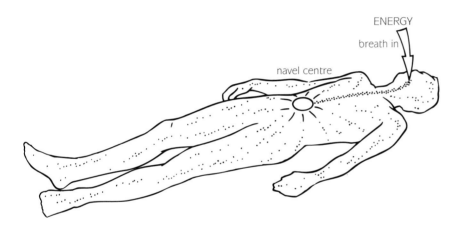

Fig. 2.3 *Relaxation with deep abdominal breathing while lying down. Visualise inward flow of energy with in-breath and energy radiating from navel throughout body on out-breath*

You can tap into this reservoir when needed. Sometimes it takes strength and determination on the part of the therapist to see a client through to better well-being, to keep up the support and guidance when it may frankly seem easier to let them go. I experienced this recently with one client. Aided by reflexology treatments and her own initiatives, she had made substantial progress but there were still several issues of health that, while not in themselves serious, were keeping her from feeling really well. It was tempting to feel that we had done enough together, but I was not satisfied and wanted to continue treatments to resolve the rest of her areas of imbalance. As she was agreeable, we continued treatments and she began to gain benefit in other areas.

1. What are the three energies that combine in the healing process?
2. Why is it important to remember that healing comes from within the client?
3. What is the difference between reacting and responding?
4. How can the therapist's self-awareness help protect both her and her clients?

Pitfalls and possibilities

Pitfalls

- The practitioner becomes the 'expert' in the situation; the client is merely the passive recipient of treatment without an active role.
- The gender of the therapist or client becomes an issue. The relationship becomes personal and does not remain professional.
- In talking with a client, the therapist may use language or terms which, while meaningful to a practitioner, are not understood by the client.
- The therapist allows their own imbalances to interfere with the treatments given; or, they allow negative energy of the client to be transferred to them.
- Focussing too much on the physical aspects of the illness and measuring improvement only on this basis, forgetting that for the physical to really improve, at some point some fundamental changes may be needed in the client's lifestyle, outlook or personal life.

GOOD PRACTICE

Respect yourself and the skills you have acquired. Have confidence in the effectiveness of reflexology.

Possibilities

- Positive communication. The practitioner actively listens to the client's experience and explains her methods in a way the client can understand (see Chapter 14).
- Mutual respect, trust and care. We respect and genuinely care for the integrity of the client. The client feels safe and in control. Compassion motivates the therapist to foster the client's own healing process. We take care not to abuse our expertise at the client's expense.
- Realistic and positive expectations. Confidence in the technique helps the client be comfortable with the treatment process. Realising its limitations means we can to refer the client to other helpers when necessary.
- Even if a condition is not fully resolved, the client gains new insights and the strength to tackle issues perhaps previously too daunting, the deeper issues that need putting right. The client has grown towards a more harmonious balance.

Key Terms

You need to know what these terms mean. Go back through the chapter or check in the glossary to find out.

- Integrity
- Vulnerability
- Breath awareness
- Transference
- Limits of training

3 THE CONSULTATION PROCESS

After working through this chapter you will be able to:

♦ understand consultation aims and procedures

♦ understand and use skills of active listening and eliciting information

♦ recognise the importance of making a clear record of a consultation and reflexology treatment

♦ recognise the need to formulate a therapeutic strategy and manage treatment sessions

♦ understand the need for observing caution when giving reflexology and know when to do so.

REMEMBER
Conducting a consultation is as much art as science. Observation and good technique are vital but equally important are intuition and the skills of good communication. See Chapter Fourteen on communication for details.

Although perhaps not obvious at first, conducting a consultation at the client's first visit and in much briefer form at subsequent visits, is one of the most important aspects of a professional reflexology practice. Taking notes and recording the consultation and treatments is a continuing process that allows us better to evaluate the effectiveness of treatments and plan future therapeutic sessions. It can also provide the raw material for research if called upon to do so. A thorough consultation enhances the effectiveness of treatments.

Aspects of a reflexology consultation include:

♦ skills in observation and communication

♦ compiling a case history

♦ recording findings of the treatment

♦ continuing to monitor and record the process of subsequent treatments consistently and accurately

♦ formulating a therapeutic strategy for treatments.

Aims of the consultation

Aims of the consultation are as follows:

♦ to observe and record factors relevant to the patient and her condition, a holistic appreciation of social, emotional, mental, and environmental factors as well as physical symptoms and appearances, medical history and any medication with which the client presents

♦ to allow the client to 'tell her own story' to an accepting audience

♦ to allow the therapist to 'tell' her story or explain the nature and efficacy of the treatment, and give further supportive advice.

At best the consultation helps foster a partnership with the mutual trust, care and respect characteristic of holistic treatment.

Confidentiality

In order for the client to feel free to be open about themselves, they need to be sure that their information will be kept absolutely confidential. Reassure them of this at the first visit. As professionals we undertake to not pass on information to another (third) party without the client's permission, although we are bound by law to report such things as instances of communicable diseases to the relevant health authorities (see page 206).

GOOD PRACTICE

Always make a record of each treatment session and keep records secure.

Progress Check

1   What are two advantages of recording the consultation and treatments?
2   What are three aims of a consultation?
3   Why is it important to assure the client of confidentiality?

Consultation skills

Active listening

Active listening could be called 'really listening'. The term is used to highlight the fact that often when talking with people we tend only to pay partial attention to what they are saying. We may be 'hearing' them but we are not listening to them in a fully receptive way. Or we might be just as keen or keener to tell them about ourselves as to share their experience. Active listening reflects that we respect the speaker because we give them the gift of our full attention.

We show our acceptance by:

- not interrupting with comments of our own
- not taking over the conversation with our own contribution, or redirecting attention to ourselves
- not being judgemental
- not changing the subject
- not switching off and allowing our minds to wander to our own concerns while the person is speaking.

Reflecting

In other words, we respond with genuine interest. When we reply, we first aim to reflect back to the speaker the essence of what we have heard her say. This reflecting phase is important because it allows the speaker to know whether we have understood her as she wanted to be understood, that her story has been heard. See Chapter 14 for details on Reflecting.

Eliciting information

Eliciting information is another aspect of the consultation which helps us focus on the client in more detail. The object here is to bring out more specific information than may have first been given. Eliciting uses open-ended questions which encourage the client to share more detail, instead of closed questions which require only a yes or no answer.

For example, if the client tells us that they have headaches, in order to understand the nature of these headaches and to discover their origin, we need to ask specific follow-up questions such as:

◆ Where in the head does it affect you? Frontal (forehead), occipital (back of head), or temporal?

Here are further examples of open-ended questions with follow-up questions:

◆ Is it in the front/back/sides/sinus area?
◆ When does it occur: mornings, before/after meals, during work, before/during/after periods, etc?
◆ What makes it worse or better: movement, rest, heat, cold?
◆ How do you usually cope with it or treat it?
◆ How long has it happened, how long does it last?
◆ Does it come on at any particular time of day or during or after an activity?
◆ How do you cope?

We are trying to discover the pattern of the condition and what sorts of things bring it on or aggravate it. The answer to a question such as 'How do you handle it?' gives us insight into how the person responds to their condition and at the same time into the mental or emotional aspects of the situation.

ACTIVITY

With a friend or fellow student, practise active listening for five minutes. Ask her to tell you about a recent experience, positive or negative. Do not compare your own similar experiences, but reflect back to them at intervals what they have told you. Ask for specific details about themselves or their experience through follow-up questions. Wait to share your own comments until they have finished and ask for your contribution. Reverse roles and practise again. Finally give feedback to each other about what it felt like to be really listened to and to have to listen fully to another.

Understanding versus prying

Getting to know our clients is not prying or idle curiosity. A therapist needs to understand the client as fully as possible, to know her 'nature' and the typical 'nature' of her ailments. Follow-up with questions to help bring out the details of the client's typical nature, her unique pattern of health and illness. Tact and sensitivity are needed and we always respect the wishes of the client if she is not ready to give us the details at that time.

Observation

This can start with the first contact with the client, which might simply be over the telephone. What can we pick up from her voice or the way she speaks that may say something about her state of mind? Does she sound nervous? confident? uncertain? Is she self-assured and articulate or a little timid and anxious?

Visual and aural clues

Observe the client for clues to her general condition and state of well-being. Make a note only if you feel any are significant. Such clues are seen in the light of the person's age, gender, occupation and so on.

You may not notice each and every one of these things in the first few minutes or even first visit, but more can be added as the consultations progress and experience is gained.

- Posture and gait, for example if one shoulder is higher than another; or if the person seems slumped or 'weighed down' with care, or if she walks easily or has a physical disability.
- Complexion and condition of the skin, hair and eyes.
- Manner of speaking, for example whether talkative, quiet, hesitant, articulate or reticent.
- Manner of dress and personal presentation: is she wrapped up against the cold, or lightly clad on a cold day?
- Breathing, for example if laboured, or appearing short of breath.
- Signs of tension in the body language, for example tightly clasped hands, stiffness, rigidity.
- Weight, if it seems appropriate for the person's height and build.

ACTIVITY

Take a short ride on a bus or train. Practise your observation skills on one or two of your fellow travellers. Notice things which seem to tell you some things about them. Their age, activity level, mannerisms, breathing, dress style. Look for things about them which may be conflicting, for example, a large brawny person who seems a little insecure, or hesitant. Based on these observations try to assess their overall state of balance.

Observing the feet

Before treatment examine the feet and record significant findings. Check such things as skin tone, texture and colour, structure, flexibility, blemishes, the temperature and moistness of the feet. Note any significant differences between left and right.

REMEMBER

What clients may not tell you verbally you can learn through your own powers of observation and intuition and the sensitivity of your hands and fingers.

All these factors are like pieces in a jigsaw puzzle that will help us work out the picture and pattern of that client's unique innate balance and any current imbalances which lie behind the condition they present with.

Some signs suggest the client's vital energy might be low. These include such things as numbness or loss of feeling, coldness, paleness, dampness or clamminess, slack muscle tone or a spongy feel to the tissues. It is also possible to sense intuitively that a person's vital energy is low.

Intuition

In the investigations above we have been using mainly our left brain faculties, our skills of rational and linear thinking. But just as important are our right brain faculties, such as intuition and creative thinking. We separate these for the sake of discussion but really we use them both all the time. Sometimes we need to listen to our intuition instead of our rational side when trying to understand what has brought the client to the present state. We may just 'get a feeling' that something is so, without as yet any rational proof – usually this emerges later.

Listening to our own intuition may not be easy for some of us, as we may not be used to trusting our own feelings. We may be used to having rational proof before we credit something. However by working with ourselves a little, learning to centre, to contact our deeper feelings and insights, and allowing them to shed their light on our understanding, we gradually gain the confidence to bring our intuition into play to more fully understand the person.

stomach, legs. At each place you ask if it is feeling OK. If you get a negative answer, such as 'neck feels really tense', acknowledge that, but put it aside for the moment as you move to another body part. As you find areas of tension, pain or excessive cold or heat, acknowledge each one and continue to check out your body until you have 'listened' and paid attention to all the parts that feel uncomfortable. If all of you is feeling well, be grateful and accept that too.

4 Choose one of your uncomfortable parts (or any part of you, if all are feeling well), think about that body part and first breathe in then lengthen the out-breath and direct it into and through that part. At the same time feel that the out-breath is taking away with it any tension or feelings of pain and discomfort. Repeat two or three times. Return to normal breathing.

5 Now notice how you feel generally. Accept it without criticism or judgement. Just be with yourself for a few moments, quietly.

6 Now choose another part of your body that felt uncomfortable. Repeat the practice of breathing into that part. Feel that as you breathe in you are taking in healing energy, as you breathe out you are directing this healing energy into and through that part of you that feels uncomfortable. Repeat this for three to five breaths, then return to normal breathing.

7 Pause to study how you feel. Notice any changes or lack of change, accepting what there is.

8 When you are ready, breathe five times into your solar plexus. As you breathe in feel the breath moving through your nostrils, down your throat, to your lungs and down to your solar plexus region. As you breathe out feel the breath radiating out from the solar plexus to all parts of your body, enlivening and energising them with the vital life force.

9 Return to normal breathing, watching the breath flow in and out. Pause to experience the deep state of calm and stillness you have discovered within you. Feel that you will act now from this calm centre of peace and strength, rather than just from your head.

10 Gradually bring yourself back to outward awareness by wiggling your toes, feet, fingers, hands. Rub your hands together. When you are ready, open your eyes. Accept what you have done and welcome what came to you. Be glad it spoke to you and you listened.

Progress Check

1 What is meant by the term 'active listening'?
2 What is the purpose of the reflecting phase of listening to someone?
3 Why is important to ask specific follow-up questions?
4 What are some possible indicators of low vital energy?
5 What types of things can we observe visually?
6 What role does intuition play in understanding?
7 What are eight indicators that you might find on a client's feet? What could each tell you about the client's health?

Record keeping

The case history and treatment record

A sample record sheet is provided with this chapter, and sample case histories are given in Appendix 2. A case history involves first recording basic personal details and then taking a case history, in which you ask the client for information about any previous medical conditions they may have experienced, including relatively minor ones if these tended to be repeated. In other words it is a health history. In addition it records pertinent information about any episode of illness.

The treatment record is a continuation of the case history into the present treatment. It is a very important activity. Here we record the findings of each reflexology treatment. Which reflexes were tender, tense, congested, perhaps noticeably cold or hot? Which reflexes changed? These details are recorded along with any particular attention given to them and the length and frequency of the treatments. This is repeated with each treatment and, as treatments continue, we can follow the progress of the client by comparing treatments with each other and with how the client is feeling.

Personal details

Although seemingly only factual and straightforward, a lot of information about the context of the client's life can be gained. For example, be attentive to the client's age and how she looks or feels compared to what you would expect (without being judgemental). Is she the major caregiver or wage earner or both? Does she work in or out of home? In a factory or office? All these things may have a bearing on the condition.

Initial observations

Observe the following and make a note only if you feel any one is significant. You may not gather all this in the first few minutes or even first visit, but more can be added as the consultations progress:

- posture
- complexion
- manner of speaking (talkative/quiet)
- manner of dress
- breathing
- signs of tension such as tightly clasped hands, stiffness, rigidity
- weight, complexion.

Complaint or inquiry

Here you ask the client to tell you why she has come, what is bothering her, what would she most like to have relief from or treatment for. The answers will vary from client to client. Often a person just wants to try out reflexology to see what it's like, or they just feel tense and in need of something to help them relax, without having any major medical or symptomatic problems.

On the other hand, many clients come with conditions for which they have received medical treatment and diagnosis, but which have not been either cured or significantly improved and they want some further help. Such conditions may be relatively minor – headaches, aches and pains – or quite serious and chronic – diabetes, arthritis, hypertension.

> **REMEMBER**
> Disturbance or imbalance in an area may suggest either emotional or otherwise stressful problems that may be a factor in the presenting condition or help explain problems already highlighted.

> **REMEMBER**
> While at first minor symptoms may not seem to have much relationship to the main condition, with time we may come to realise there is a connection.

Sometimes a person comes with one major complaint but other lesser, relatively minor ones.

Here is where we especially practise active listening, eliciting and intuition.

Medical history

Ask about:

- any past medical conditions including those of childhood
- major and minor traumas such as falls and accidents; emotional traumas (loss of a loved-one, moving home)
- any operations, hospitalisations, serious illness, allergies
- any medications both past and present
- any major diseases in the family: heart or circulatory (e.g. phlebitis), kidney, liver, respiratory, nervous (e.g. epilepsy), metabolic (e.g. diabetes).

REMEMBER
Ask follow-up questions to discover if an episode was successfully resolved or may have left some remnant of imbalance, either emotional or physical. If the client is reluctant to disclose details, accept this at this time.

Systems assessment

Briefly check the functioning of each system of the body. This check helps us to:

- pick up information the client may forget to mention
- from a holistic point of view, to discover how the different systems are functioning in relation to each other, where the imbalances are likely to be. This can be compared to findings on the feet
- understand how the conditions the client presents with may have come about
- understand how the condition is affecting the rest of the body, both emotional-mental and physical.

REMEMBER
It is not necessary to ask each question given below, they are suggestions only. Some reflexologists prefer to wait until the treatment and ask such questions as and when tender areas come up in each area considered.

Appetite and digestion

Ask how the appetite is to discover if the appetite is good (enjoys food and eating), poor (avoids/ skips, indifferent, erratic), or excessive. Ask if there is any disturbance to good digestion such as: heartburn, acidity, aches, headaches with eating, marked flatulence, cramps.

Diet

Ask for a typical day's diet, from rising to bedtime, including drinks and snacks. This will give you a good idea of the client's overall pattern and might point out areas of imbalance. To save time, you may request the client to supply you with this in writing for the next visit.

Bowels

Don't be shy of asking about this area and educating your clients of its importance. However, handle the subject with sensitivity. If the client seems reluctant, move on; otherwise ask such questions as: how do your bowels move? Once a day or more or less often? Do you ever suffer from diarrhoea or constipation? Haemorrhoids? Cramps? Other? If the client mentions blood in the stool advise referral to GP for check-up.

REMEMBER
Appetite and good digestion are fundamental to good health. No matter how high the quality of the food we eat, if digestion is poor we cannot derive the nutrition and energy we need from it. Eating patterns are good indicators of overall health.

Urinary

Ask about any history of problems in this area, for example, cystitis, urinary tract infection and any medication taken; any pressure or pain on passing urine. If the client mentions blood in the urine, advise referral to GP for check-up.

Respiratory

Ask about any problems here, for example, sinus, short breath, allergies, frequent colds, flu or coughing, ear infections; history of bronchitis or other problems and medication taken.

Lymphatic

Ask if the client has ever experienced swelling in the glands: cervical, axilla, breasts, groin; if there is history of tonsillitis or tonsils removed, swollen adenoids, frequent infections or not fully recovered from an infection, still feeling tired.

Skin

Ask about history of any skin problems, for example, skin allergies, eczema, dry skin. Observe for yourself and perhaps only enquire if you have noticed anything.

Circulatory

Ask about history of varicose veins, chilblains, blood pressure or heart problems. Does the client 'feel the cold', or alternatively does she usually feel hot or stuffy.

Musculo-skeletal

Ask about history of injuries, fractures, traumas, aches or pains in the bones, muscles or joints.

Nervous and endocrine

Ask about headaches, tension, spasms, pains, moods and whether there is overall good immunity. This area overlaps that below on the emotional-mental state, and stress factors.

Reproductive system

This area may require extra tact and sensitivity.

- Ask women about the pattern of their period, if it is particularly painful, heavy or scant; if there are signs of pre-menstrual syndrome (if before a period there is bloating, cramps, fatigue, headaches, irritability or moodiness, any one or all of these). Ask about the menarche, any traumas or trouble associated with it? As appropriate for older women, ask about how the menopause is or was for them, any problems and how they dealt with them.
- Men from the age of 40 may begin to have prostate problems. However before that age you can just ask in a general way if there are any problems in this area and leave open the possibility that the client may tell you about any other problem such as impotence, without you directly asking about it.

Life-style assessment

Here ask about or make a note if the client mentions the following:

- lifestyle (very active/sedentary, overworks, unemployed, etc.)
- food preferences: hot/spicy, sweets and puddings, vegetarian, savoury, wholefood?
- eating habits such as 'always eats on the go', or skips meals often, or likes three 'square' meals a day; exercise, such as what type, if any, how often; if no or little exercise taken, why?
- relaxation and recreation.

Recreation is an important, often overlooked area, which allows us to switch off from demands and purely enjoy ourselves. Afterwards, we can often cope with other distressing circumstances better.

REMEMBER
Relaxation allows the body to repair and recover itself.

Emotional-mental factors

It is difficult asking about emotional factors, especially at the initial consultation when trust is just beginning to be established. Rather than doing so directly, we can infer it from what the client tells us in any item above and from asking about sleep, energy and stress.

Sleep
Ask about the client's sleep pattern. If there is a problem, ask follow up questions such as: is sleep often/sometimes interrupted; can she easily get back to sleep; does she wake up refreshed or tired?

General energy level
Does she feel she has enough energy for what she wants to do; or does she start off with energy but soon run out; or does she tire easily, or feel tired often?

Stress
Is the client under any particular stress in the home, at work; around relationships with relatives or friends or colleagues? How well is the client coping? Does she feel supported when going through difficulties or not?

REMEMBER
Disturbance or imbalance in either of these areas may suggest either emotional or physical problems that may be a factor in the presenting condition or help explain problems already highlighted. They can also suggest ways in which you can help the client indirectly even when you cannot directly treat for a condition.

ACTIVITY
Take a case history of yourself. Record it in your health journal. Once you have finished, think about what you have recorded and reflect on your own health patterns, the health of each of your systems and your strengths and weaknesses in terms of health. What sort of ailments, if any, do you seem predisposed to? Do you see an overall positive or negative pattern in your health history? What steps can you take to improve or maintain your health?

GOOD PRACTICE

Explain briefly to the client the need to ask questions for the case history. Be sensitive, tactful and discreet. Reassure the client of the confidentiality of the information.

Progress Check

1 What is the purpose of taking a case history?
2 Why might it be important to record medications taken, and operations?
3 Why is it helpful to understand the diet of the client?
4 What can sleep patterns tell us about overall health?

Recording the reflexology treatment

Record each treatment given on a record sheet. A suggested format is given, but you may change or adapt this to your own style. Record in brief note form, using clear abbreviations.

1 Record any observations of obvious significance about the feet such as temperature, differences between left and right, skin tone and condition, abrasions, warts, corns, calluses.
2 Record any cautions you will observe in treatment.
3 At each treatment after the first one, record briefly the client's response to the previous treatment. Was there any improvement, if so how and where? If the client experienced no noticeable improvement note this as well. Try to use some of the client's own words if possible.
4 As you give the treatment, record the client's responses as the treatment progresses. You can do this either pictorially or in written form, as shown. It is good to devise a code and stick with it. For example use a 'T' for very tender areas, a 't' for less tender areas, a 'c' for areas that are not tender to the client but reveal tissue congestion to your touch, 'ts' for tension. Alternatively you may use different coloured inks, such as red, blue, green. The important thing is to note what symbols or colours mean, and to be consistent. This way when you look back on a case you can understand what you have recorded.

GOOD PRACTICE

Observe carefully. Record accurately. Think creatively. Listen to your own intuitions.

If you use the written form of record keeping you will need also to record the location reflexes accurately. It's a good idea to use a system of general areas divided by the landmarks and the zones, and to divide these into upper, middle, lower.

Reflex record no.
Name:
Date:

Observations	Right foot	Left foot
	Right foot	Left foot
Diaphragm		
Head/sinus/neck		Ⓣ cervicles T-1
Chest/lungs/heart		
Lymph, clavicle		
Stomach	ⓣ upper zone 2	
Pancreas		
Liver	Ⓒ	
Spleen		
Large intestine		
Small intestine		
Sigmoid		
Bladder		
Kidney		
Adrenal		
Thyroid/parathyroid		
Pituitary		
Reproductive		
Lymph groin		
Spine		
Muscle-skeleton (shoulder, knees etc)	hip, lateral Ⓣ	

T = very tender   t = slightly tender   Recommendations:
c = congestion   ts = tension   Next treatment
                                            date:
                                            Therapeutic strategy:

Fig. 3.1 *(a) A record sheet (chart format) for recording treatments and showing how the location of a tender reflex could be recorded*

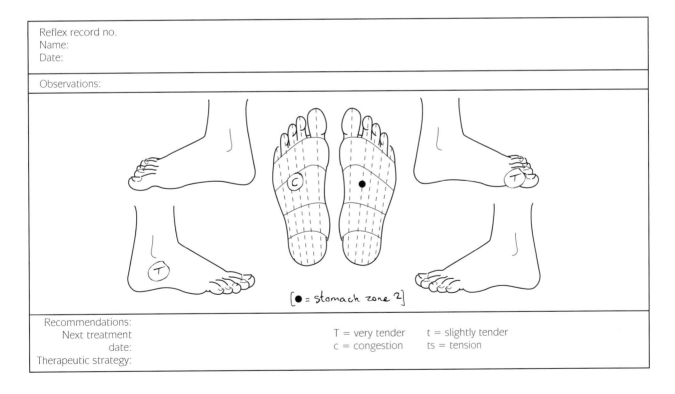

Reflex record no.
Name:
Date:

Observations:

[● = stomach zone 2]

Recommendations:
Next treatment
date: T = very tender   t = slightly tender
Therapeutic strategy: c = congestion   ts = tension

Fig. 3.1 *(b) A record sheet (drawing format) for recording treatments including an example of the location of a tender reflex on a grid*

For example, a tender area may be in the stomach area, zone 2, but nearer the diaphragm than the waistline, hence at the stomach line, record ' t, upper z-2'. For the pelvic or spinal areas be as accurate as you can in recording the exact reflex area, for example, 'pelvic area, lateral'.

If using pictures, you can create a grid with landmarks and zone lines and indicate tender reflexes on this.

With either system, you can then tell if the exact area is tender at the next treatment.

5   At the end of the treatment:
   ♦   record any important observations you notice about the client or which she tells you. For example, her general level of sensitivity or tension – was the client more relaxed afterwards? Did she drift into sleep? Record words she used to describe her feelings, such as 'I feel like I'm floating', 'The pain in my head is better', 'I feel a twinge in my knee'
   ♦   record any intuitions you have if significant
   ♦   record any precautions you observed during the treatment.

The therapeutic strategy

Formulating a therapeutic strategy means defining objectives for your treatments and how best to approach the client. It helps to focus assessment on the weakest areas that need the most support in terms of reflexology – which systems are most in need of the cleansing, balancing, or stimulating effects of reflexology – and recording these from treatment to treatment.

Although you will be treating the whole foot you will also be concentrating on specific areas of treatment. Your therapeutic strategy cannot really be formed after the verbal consultation, for you also rely enormously on 'what the feet can tell' as Eunice Ingham recognised. But even at this point you can begin to get an idea based on the case history and then you can compare this with what you find through the feet. Sometimes the feet will seem to tell a different story – not confirming your intuitions, or what the client has told you, which can be puzzling. Don't be discouraged, but keep an open mind and remember that this is the initial consultation and it often takes time for the true situation to be revealed. Form a 'working strategy' and be prepared to change it if necessary.

It is important to record your initial strategy even if you subsequently change your mind about it and revise it. This is a creative, on-going process of revision in the light of any changes that occur, any new information that is revealed, any insights. We, as therapists, are open to the healing power of nature as revealed in each client.

At the second and subsequent treatments you will also record how the client responds to the treatments. With the information you receive verbally from the client, from your own observations and intuitions and from what the feet reveal, you form the strategy for subsequent treatments.

Recommendations

Here record such things as:

- further treatments you recommend , for example: weekly for three weeks then reassess
- any advice you may give to the client, for example: to take more exercise, to work on their own reflexes, to take a vitamin supplement, to see the GP. Whatever it is, record it here. At the next visit, ask if they have followed up your suggestions.

After the treatment itself, you help your client off the couch, if used, to a seated position. At this time discuss your most significant findings with the client, answer any questions and make your recommendations verbally. The main point is to explain what you are doing and how you interpret the findings to the client. Some discussion of the reflexes will usually occur during treatment, but at this time you can summarise them again.

Also give general aftercare advice such as to drink a little extra water to aid the cleansing process which has been initiated with the treatment and to take extra rest if possible. You can explain to the client about the possibility, though not inevitability, of a 'healing crisis', what it means, and how she should interpret it and respond.

Before closing the session, agree with the client about follow-up treatments. Give your assessment as to whether the client would benefit, the length of sessions, how many and how often you recommend treatment. Negotiate with the client what is needed and what is manageable for her.

> **REMEMBER**
> Keep good verbal and eye contact with the client, watching her face in order to gauge the effect of your pressure.

Follow-up treatments and managing treatment sessions

At subsequent treatments you will be repeating some aspects of the initial consultation in order to monitor progress: you continue to inquire about the client's health and as necessary, the functioning of various systems, to see if there has been improvement or not. Check particularly those aspects that you are treating for. As you give treatment, continue to 'listen' to what the feet have to tell you and to your own intuitions. Record which treatment areas are emphasised, and if there is any change, or not, to the reflexes. Note any new symptoms or changes in the condition of the feet.

At each new treatment session, again record the date, length and overall conduct of the session. Ask how the client has responded to the previous treatment and record any feedback, whether the results seem positive and the client felt better, or negative and the client experienced some negative symptoms or responses. Responses can include emotions or changes in attitudes or lifestyle, as well as changes in physical signs, or the presenting condition. Record these, keeping an open mind. Record your new therapeutic strategy for the next session, which reflexes you expect to be emphasising or monitoring especially carefully.

> **REMEMBER**
> Often the full effects of reflexology are cumulative and sometimes not seen for four or more treatments, depending on the client and the condition. It is helpful to encourage the client to commit to at least four sessions, then the situation can be reassessed and changes made accordingly.

Negative reactions

Don't be discouraged if things seem to go backward for a while; this may be a necessary part of the healing process. Eunice Ingham found that often reflexes became more tender with the third or fourth treatments but her experience showed her that this was a positive sign. It showed the vital force was returning to these areas and activating their functions to a higher level, hence they were more sensitive. Keep a calm and open mind, waiting for the body to respond.

After enquiring about the response, give the treatment and record the sensitivities as you find them and your observations and recommendations at the end of the treatment.

Progress Check

1   How can keeping clear records of a case help you in your work?
2   How is it helpful to check through the functioning of the different systems with the client before treatment? Why might some reflexologists prefer not to do this?
3   How can forming a therapeutic strategy help focus the treatment?
4   Why is it important to record any recommendations you make to a client?

Contra-indications or cautions for reflexology

The question of cautions or contra-indications for reflexology is somewhat controversial. Different leaders in the field have different approaches. Generally the approach of Ingham's teachings is that there are virtually no contra-indications because reflexology is so inherently safe; any stimulation is done at a distance and is very gentle.

However, it is also the case that complementary medicine in general does not yet enjoy the general approval of society at large and the medical establishment in particular. So for the practitioner's own protection as much as the client's, certain precautions may need to be observed.

Some reflexologists prefer to use the criteria of 'caution', feeling 'contra-indication' is too absolute and unnecessary. Each client and their condition needs to be assessed individually and, treatment will vary according to the skill, experience and expertise of the reflexologist. In practice, treatment for one client may be appropriate while for another it is not, even though they have been diagnosed as having the same medical condition. In other words, the client is treated holistically. Also treatment can always be adapted to the individual and their condition. This is an example where the holistic approach is different from the conventional medical one.

When in doubt about whether to treat or not, give a general treatment, leaving out problematic areas until further advice can be obtained from the client's doctor or a more experienced reflexologist. Discuss with the client the best way to proceed for her. Work within your limits of experience and training.

Suggested cautions

The following approaches to precautions indicate the range of positions taken on this issue. Ultimately each therapist must make up his or her own mind.

Franz Wagner lists the following conditions as unsuitable for treatment:

- infectious diseases
- acute fevers
- inflammations of the venous and lymphatic systems
- conditions requiring surgery
- diseases or conditions of the foot which make treatment impossible, for example, major skin problems.

Laura Norman finds that it is a good idea to treat fevers if a brief, light treatment is given and directed to glands and the liver to aid detoxification.

Other teachers caution on:

- heavy periods
- tachycardia – avoid the heart area
- shingles – wait until the rash has gone
- continued extreme negative reaction to treatment
- internal bleeding
- gangrene
- first trimester of pregnancy
- lymphatic cancer
- phlebitis.

Anna Kaye cautions no treatment:

- if the patient is under heavy drug medication; Kaye reasons that a cleansing reaction may result, eliminating the drug from the system more quickly than would occur otherwise. Also the purposes of the two would be in conflict
- after internal surgery until the doctor has pronounced complete recovery.

Doreen Bayly, who studied with Eunice Ingham before teaching reflexology in Britain, lists no contra-indications but adds the following cautions:

- use light pressure when treating children, who are more responsive and reactive
- in cases of chronic heart trouble, treat the heart reflex more carefully – lightly, gently, sensitively, and only briefly – until the general condition of the whole body has responded to the work and muscle tone improved
- cases of thrombosis should be referred to the GP for approval.

> **REMEMBER**
> Even when a condition of the foot, such as an injury, strain or local skin condition prevents treatment, the hands may be used instead. This is the versatility of reflexology.

Inge Dougans also gives cautions:

- deep vein thrombosis because of the possibility of stimulating the blood clot to detach and migrate to another part of the body, for example brain or heart
- diabetes, especially insulin-dependent type, because of the possibility of stimulating the pancreas to produce insulin which would add to that received by injection, thus upsetting the blood sugar balance. Again, discussing the treatment with the GP before commencing is a good idea so the situation can be monitored.

Follow the advice of medical practitioners

As reflexology grows in popularity and is practised more widely, for example in nursing homes, or hospitals, drug addiction clinics, and on psychiatric patients, many more situations will occur which need to be judged individually, with discrimination and sensitivity, and the advice of doctors and nurses in charge followed.

It may be wise to obtain the doctor's advice after a client has surgery. However, many reflexologists and their clients have found that having reflexology before surgery helps to minimise the negative effects of the trauma to the body and helps the body recover sooner. Treatment commenced soon after surgery also speeds recovery.

Consult with the client

Even very experienced reflexologists do not always agree on these topics. Whenever there is any doubt or cause for concern, discuss the subject with the client and together agree on the therapeutic approach. This too should be recorded in the case notes. It is possible to give a treatment leaving out any controversial areas. The client will still receive enormous benefit from the reflexology.

A general guideline is that as a therapist, you take into consideration all the factors:

- the client holistically: her nature, current state, degree of sensitivity
- the nature of the ailment or imbalances
- your own level of experience and expertise
- any medications the client is on
- the advice of the client's doctor if relevant.

ACTIVITY

With fellow students, your teacher or other reflexologists, draw up a list of conditions and situations in which you would first pause for thought before deciding on treatment. Discuss the pros and cons of each between yourselves. Discuss the meaning of the term 'within the limits of training'.

1   What is the difference between a caution and a contra-indication?

2   Why might treating a person with a deep vein thrombosis be problematic?

3   Why is it important to follow the advice of medical professionals when treating clients in hospitals?

4   How might reflexology have an effect on a client's medication, for example insulin?

Key Terms

You need to know what these terms mean. Go back through the chapter or check in the glossary to find out.

- Active listening
- Open-ended questions
- Cautions
- Intuition
- Record keeping
- Eliciting
- Closed questions
- Therapeutic strategy
- Contra-indications
- Case history

After working through this chapter you will be able to:

- understand the importance of creating a therapeutic space for clients
- recognise the importance of the setting of the treatment
- recognise the importance of the client's comfort and security
- understand the variety of positions in which treatment can be given which allow good communication
- understand the furnishings and basic equipment needed to give treatment
- recognise the requirements of first aid, safety, hygiene and access
- understand the process in the therapeutic space.

In seeking to create the conditions which allow the client's own innate healing force to come into play, the physical environment in which the reflexology treatment is given can play an important role. The reflexology treatment session comprises a distinct period of time and an environment – a 'therapeutic space' – in which the client feels safe and relaxed enough to be open to the healing process. Such a space is like an oasis of tranquility among the stresses and turbulence of life's demands.

Many factors contribute to this environment and this chapter will look at a range of them. Although the settings of a treatment may vary with the client and the reflexologist, many factors can be accommodated in most settings.

GOOD PRACTICE

Create within yourself a calm, centred space from which you give treatments. Develop the intention and ability to be 'present' with the client, as a vehicle or catalyst for the healing process, giving treatment in a supporting, non-judgemental, empathising way.

Practicalities

Giving careful consideration to the nature of the physical surroundings is important. Whether the treatments take place at a clinic, in the client's home, in an office, a hospital or a room in the therapist's house, the atmosphere we try to create is a relaxed but caring one of calmness, clarity, positivity.

Reflexology is inherently a very simple technique. Strictly speaking, all that is really necessary are the hands of the therapist and the client's willingness to give feet or hands. However, in a professional setting certain arrangements are advisable.

Setting

Ensure the setting is clean, well-ventilated and heated, with some natural light. The ability to adjust the room temperature to some extent is helpful because many clients are cold or might become cooler as they relax, while others are more warm natured. The room should be well-maintained and have a welcoming, positive, relaxing atmosphere and decor.

If working in a hospital or health club setting, ensure a minimum of privacy with screens.

Entry to a clinic, or therapy room in the home should be kept freely accessible and safe for the clients. Wheelchair access should be available.

Dress and grooming

The style of dress you adopt for reflexology is an individual matter but a professional appearance is valuable. Some reflexologists like to wear a tunic, others a long white shirt or coat to lend an air of distinction or professionalism. This may be especially appropriate when working in a hospital or similar settings. Others find this creates a barrier between them and the client, and prefer to dress more informally but neatly. The important factor is good grooming which creates a positive impression, enhances confidence and reflects a professional approach.

Hair is to be kept neatly out of the way of treatment. Hands should be washed between each client. Nails need to be kept very short and clean. Rings, watches and dangling jewellery should be removed when giving treatment.

> **REMEMBER**
> Our overall aim is to promote and enhance the client's self-healing energies.

GOOD PRACTICE

Ensure the client's comfort and security and also your own.

Equipment and furnishings

The aim here is to see to the client's comfort and to enhance the therapeutic atmosphere. Keep a supply of blankets, thick towels and cushions available to ensure the client is comfortably warm and that head, neck and limbs are supported. Support under the knees is especially important to take any strain off the lower back. Use a cushion or rolled up towel for this. A box of tissues comes in handy for a variety of occasions.

Treatment chairs

Some reflexologists give treatments with the client sitting in a comfortable chair or recliner while the therapist sits on a lower chair or stool. A portable chiropodists' type support for the client's legs and feet is useful. It is also important to ensure the chair for you, the practitioner, also gives good support and allows you to move freely. It should be of a height that allows you to be comfortable while working the feet, with the hands about chest height. Remember that you may be giving treatments throughout a day and need to protect yourself against repetitive strain

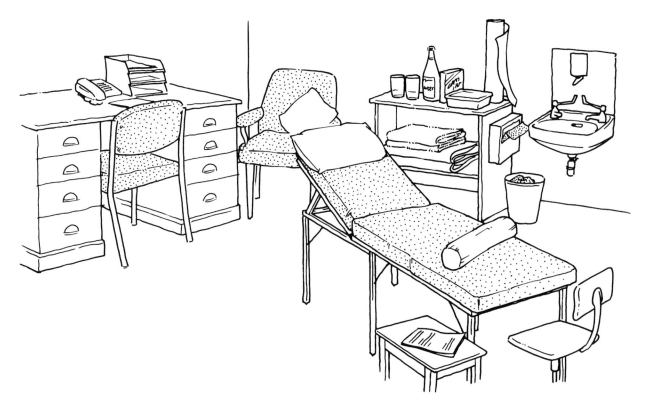

Fig. 4.1 *(a) A treatment room furnished with couch and accessories*

injury which may occur if your arms are either too high or too low. A chair or stool with an adjustable seat and wheels can be very useful to help you to vary your position as needed and adjust to the client's position.

Treatment couches

Some reflexologists prefer to have the client lying on a massage-type couch. However, if possible, the client's head and upper body are best raised, either with cushions or ideally by a couch with a moveable part that lifts up the back and head. This prevents strain on the client's lower back and allows the vital eye contact and communication which is a hallmark of reflexology. For home visits a portable recliner may be a possibility.

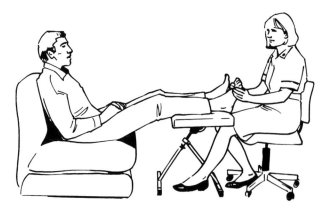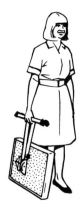

Fig. 4.1 *(b) A mini-couch is ideal for reflexology, clinic or home visits, shown here in use and as a portable item carried by the therapist*

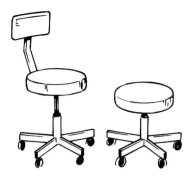

Fig. 4.1 *(c) Types of stool useful for reflexology*

If using a treatment couch it is a good idea to cover it with a sheet. Many reflexologists like to use paper from a couch roll for clients to lie on.

Music
Some reflexologists like to work with a quiet background of relaxing music. Others find this distracting for themselves and the client as it hinders the client being 'present' in the treatment. You may ask the client for her preference. (See *Performing rights* on page 204.)

Additional equipment
A small desk or table and a file for your papers, or a portfolio when making home visits. Any file or filing cabinet should be kept secure to protect confidentiality.

Comfortable chairs for the consultation, if desired.

Cornflour may be used to lubricate the feet as necessary. It is better than talc because the particles do not irritate the respiratory passages and enter the body as easily. It is preferable to using massage oil because oil tends to over-lubricate, making it easier for the fingers to skip over the pressure points. Some reflexologists like to use a cream for lubrication.

Having a bottle of spring water and glasses on hand is a good idea so clients may have a drink after treatment if they wish.

> **REMEMBER**
> See to your client's comfort at all times and be sure you can comfortably see the client's face to allow the good communication and eye contact which is vital to the treatment.

Hygiene
Ensure there are facilities for washing your hands. Professional clinics should have a wash basin available with antiseptic soap and paper towels. If this is not possible in other settings, have a stock of antiseptic wet-wipes or surgical spirit. The client's feet should be cleaned before treatment. The practitioner's hands should be cleaned before and after each treatment.

Toilet and washing facilities should be available for clients' use. Clients often appreciate the use of a mirror too.

Aftercare
We should be able to offer our clients a drink of water or a cup of tea after treatment and, if possible, a place to sit for a moment before leaving. Water helps the cleansing process begun with the treatment and should be advised for all clients. This also helps reinforce the advice to take time to care for themselves. If treatments are given in the client's home or a hospital, a bottle of water and paper cups can be carried.

> **REMEMBER**
> The lives of many people are rushed and stressful. Try to provide an oasis of tranquility for your clients which relieves some of the strain and nourishes their inner well-being.

Progress Check

1 What is the intention behind creating a therapeutic space?
2 What is as important, or even more important, than the physical setting?
3 What are some disadvantages and advantages of having background music playing during treatments?
4 What safety precautions do you need to consider for the place of your practice?
5 What hygiene considerations must you implement for your clients and yourself?
6 What are the disadvantages of using talc and cream for giving treatments?

Safety

First aid

When working from your home, in a clinic, or travelling to a client's residence, a first aid box should be available, equipped and kept up to date. To comply with the Health and Safety (First-Aid) Regulations 1981 and the revised Approved Code of Practice 2 July 1990, most reflexologists will require the following as minimum in their first aid box:

- guidance card explaining how to use the contents
- 20 individually wrapped sterile adhesive dressings
- 2 sterile eye pads, no. 16
- 6 individually wrapped triangular bandages, preferably sterile
- a pair of disposable gloves
- 6 safety pins
- 6 medium sterile unmedicated wound dressings, no. 8 or 13
- 2 large sterile unmedicated wound dressings, no. 9, 14 or amb. no. 1
- 3 extra large unmedicated wound dressings, amb. no. 3.

In addition, soap, water and disposable drying materials should be available for first aid purposes. Where soap and water cannot be available, individually wrapped, moist cleansing wipes which are not impregnated with alcohol may be used. The use of antiseptics is not necessary for treating wounds. It is also a good idea to keep a stock of sugar lumps or sweet biscuits on hand in case a client has an emergency hypoglycaemic attack.

Sterile water or normal sterile saline solution should be available in sealed disposable containers for eye irrigation in cases where mains tap water is not available; 900ml should be provided and each container should hold at least 300ml and should never be re-used once the seal is broken. Do not use eye cups, baths, or refillable containers for eye irrigation.

The travelling first aid kit
This should contain the following:

- guidance card explaining how to use the contents
- 6 individually wrapped sterile adhesive dressings
- 2 triangular bandages
- 2 safety pins
- 1 large sterile unmedicated wound dressing, no. 9, 14 or amb. no.1
- individually wrapped, moist cleansing wipes
- a pair of disposable gloves.

ACTIVITY

Research and make notes on the appropriate first aid response to the following events which may occur in your clinic:

nose bleed   faint   asthma attack

Risk assessments
First aid trainers recommend that a risk assessment should be carried out on the premises to minimise the risk of accidents. The idea is to think ahead about what could go wrong and how you can make emergencies easier to deal with. Some questions you might consider include:

- is access into and out of the premises safe?
- is it easy to get an ambulance to the site?
- are the premises well sign-posted?
- what is the grid reference on local maps?
- is the telephone always in working order?

Emergency action
In the event of an emergency, the following procedure is recommended if you are on your own.

1 Assess the scene
Obtain help if needed by telephoning 999. With help coming or delayed proceed as follows and use the ABC procedure. ABC stands for Airway, Breathing, and Circulation.

- Make the area safe for everyone.
- Check for injuries, remove all potential sources of injury.
- Reassess at intervals.

2 Assess the casualty
- Check if conscious by shaking or shouting.
- A: check the airway. Remove any obvious obstructions. Open with chin lift and head tilt.

REMEMBER
ABC stands for Airway, Breathing, Circulation.

- B: check breathing by looking, listening and feeling for 5 seconds.
- C: check circulation by feeling the pulse in the neck for 5 seconds.

3 Act on assessment
- If breathing with pulse but unconscious, place in the recovery position, and continue to monitor until help arrives. The recovery position helps airways to remain open, prevents the tongue blocking the throat yet allows vomit or liquid to drain from the mouth.
- If not breathing but with pulse, then open and clear the airway and give resuscitation as trained.
- If not breathing and there is no pulse, open and clear the airway and start chest compression or cardio-pulmonary resuscitation as trained.

GOOD PRACTICE

Keep your first aid skills intact by taking refresher training every year.

In the case of a client having an epileptic seizure
- Do nothing but remove any danger to the person from items in the area.
- When the client has come out of the seizure, ask if this is her first fit and if yes, call an ambulance by dialling 999. If not ask, how you may further assist her.

In the case of an asthma attack
- Ask if this is more than a normal attack and if yes, call an ambulance by dialling 999.
- If no, ask if the client wants to go to hospital and assist.

REMEMBER
Keep calm and follow procedures as trained.

In the case of an attack of hypoglycaemia
You may notice or the client may complain of one or more of the following: weakness or faintness, hunger, palpitations, confusion or loss of consciousness, sweating, pallor, cold, clammy skin, a bounding pulse, shallow breathing, violent or strange behaviour.

Help the client to lie or sit down and give them a sugary drink (fruit juice) or food (sugar lump or sweet biscuit). As the condition improves you can give more sweet food or drink. Allow the client to rest until fully recovered and advise a visit to the doctor.

ACTIVITY

With a group of fellow students discuss how you might react to emergency situations. Express your concerns and listen and learn from each other's experiences.

1 Why is it a good idea to carry out a risk assessment before you set up your practice? How often would you review this assessment?
2 Find out about local first aid training courses: how often they are run and by whom, what is involved.
3 What should be the contents of a first aid box?
4 What does ABC stand for?
5 What are the objectives of the recovery position?

The process in the therapeutic space

If we put together the essence of the discussions of this and previous chapters, we can form a model for the process that occurs during a reflexology session. We can visualise the therapeutic relationship and therapeutic space as a Circle of Healing created for the client.

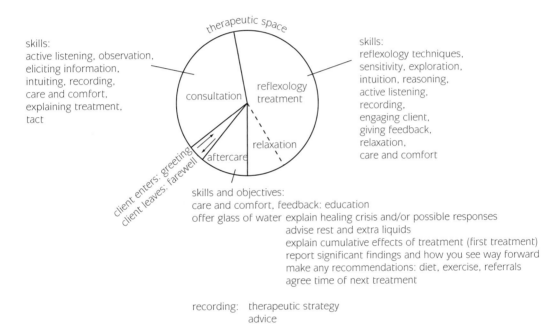

Fig. 4.2 *The process of treatment within therapeutic space*

First stage: greeting
The client enters and you make initial contact, greeting and introducing yourself. If the client is new to reflexology, explain what reflexology involves or answer any questions, and make her feel at ease.

Second stage: consultation
This is where the consultation begins – listening to the complaint, taking the medical history and systems details. Here active listening, eliciting and recording skills are in play. Respond with a caring attitude and begin to process the information you are receiving.

Third stage: treatment
Now the treatment itself begins with making the client comfortable, observing the feet and giving general relaxation techniques. As you

proceed with treating the reflexes record your findings, maintain communication with the client visually and verbally and work with her as needed. Allow relaxation time at the end of the treatment; while the client is quiet, finish your notes, recording your therapeutic strategy and what recommendations you will be making, if any.

Fourth stage: aftercare and closing

When the client has risen from the couch and/or is sitting comfortably, you give aftercare.

- Offer the client a glass of water and advise her to drink extra water over the next 24 hours to enhance the cleansing process.
- Advise her to rest as much as possible to enhance the effects of the treatment.
- Discuss with the client any significant findings from the feet, relating these to her condition.
- Explain possible responses to the treatment some clients may experience, such as mild tiredness or headaches. Discuss this within the context of explaining the healing crisis, emphasising that if discomfort is experienced it is likely to be the result of positive healing activity in the body.
- Explain the cumulative effects of reflexology treatments – the fact that the greatest benefits may take three or more treatments to be noticed, as it may take time for any patterns of imbalanced energy flow to be altered. Also point out that some people naturally respond quickly to treatment, others take a little longer.
- Answer any questions and also make any recommendations about further treatments, diet or lifestyle changes, and referrals if necessary. This rounds off and closes the session and the client leaves.

Within this circle of time you have endeavoured to give your client your best attention and care, confident in the healing power of reflexology – a vital, healing human touch.

Within this circle the client has benefited from a space of time all to herself where she was able to relax deeply, taking time to allow her body to balance and be supported as it heals itself with its own vital force.

Key Terms

You need to know what these terms mean. Go back through the chapter or check in the glossary to find out.

- Therapeutic space
- Being present
- Closing
- ABC
- Tranquility
- Catalyst
- Recovery position

Further reading

Mitchell, A. and Cormak, M. *The Therapeutic Relationship in Health Care*. Churchill Livingstone, London. 1998.

After working through this chapter you will be able to:

♦ understand the zone paradigm as lines of energy flow
♦ understand the anatomical correspondences between feet and body
♦ understand holistic correspondences between feet and body
♦ read and use the map of the feet to locate reflexes and know the reasons for variations in some maps
♦ understand how the feet can reflect the body
♦ understand some of the conditions of the feet and how these reflect the body's health.

Modern reflexology was derived from Zone Therapy developed by Dr William Fitzgerald. His work helped to show that different parts of the body relate to and influence one another at an energetic level along longitudinal zones, as well as a physiological one via the nerves and circulation. An energetic approach helps us see that the human body is more than just a mechanical machine with different parts working together. The mechanical model obscures the fact that this is a living organism whose various parts and systems have the ability to constantly communicate with, relate to and influence each other and the whole.

The zone paradigm: lines of energy flow

In Fitzgerald's zone paradigm we can see how the organs and systems relate to each other. Of special note is the fact that on each big toe each of the five zones for that side of the body also flow. We also note that organs in the same zone can affect each other via the zones. For example, we find that the kidneys and the eyes lie in the same zones, 2 and 3, and empirical experience with reflexology has shown over the years that often eye problems go with signs of kidney weakness in many people. Similarly, some headaches show on the feet not only with tenderness in the head reflex areas but also in the lower bowel reflexes in the same zone lines, showing that an imbalance in the lower bowel is affecting the head, and may even be the root cause of the headache.

This information can help guide the reflexologist to find the underlying cause of a particular symptom by noting any sensitivity in other organs within the same zone lines of energy, and working on these reflexes as well. By treating the root cause as well as the symptom site, we effect a better resolution of the problem.

> **REMEMBER**
> The zone lines as illustrated are symbolic. In reality each zone spans more than a single line. It takes in a longitudinal area of the body.

The feet reflect the person
There are many ways the feet reflect the rest of the body. Their structure and condition, as well as the individual reflexes, can tell us much about the client's condition and history.

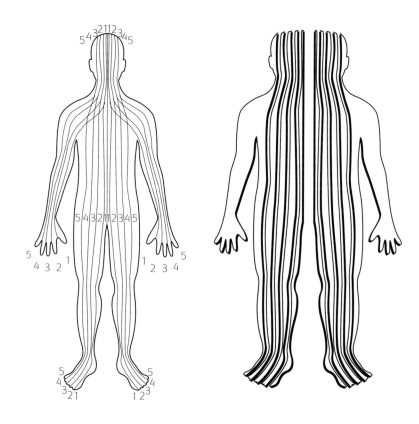

Fig. 5.1 *(a) Illustration showing zones as three-dimensional sections of the body*

Anatomy of the foot

The foot is made up of: bones, muscles, ligaments, tendons, skin, blood vessels and nerves. Its functions are to support the weight of the body and, co-ordinated with the action of the legs, to propel the body or lever it off the ground.

There are 26 bones in the foot: seven tarsal bones, five metatarsal bones and fourteen phalanges. The calcaneus and the talus bear the weight of the body onto the foot, The tarsals and metatarsals together support the arches of the foot.

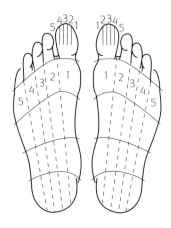

Fig. 5.1 *(b) Zone areas on the feet. Note that all five zones are found on the big toe and each small toe repeats and 'magnifies' the zone of the relevant head area.*

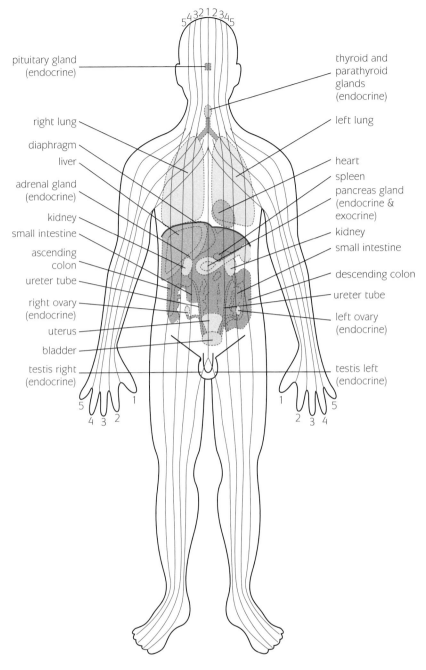

pituitary gland (endocrine)

thyroid and parathyroid glands (endocrine)

right lung

left lung

diaphragm

liver

heart

spleen

adrenal gland (endocrine)

pancreas gland (endocrine & exocrine)

kidney

kidney

small intestine

small intestine

ascending colon

descending colon

ureter tube

ureter tube

right ovary (endocrine)

left ovary (endocrine)

uterus

bladder

testis right (endocrine)

testis left (endocrine)

Fig. 5.1 *(c) Schematic diagram indicating placement of major organs and glands within zone lines*

There are three arches in the foot:

- the medial, or inner longitudinal arch
- the lateral or outer longitudinal arch
- the transverse arch.

The toes are supported by the phalanges, two in the halux or big toe, and three in each of the other toes. The structure of the foot can influence its condition as can the health of the other tissues, particularly the musculature and circulation (see pages 76–80).

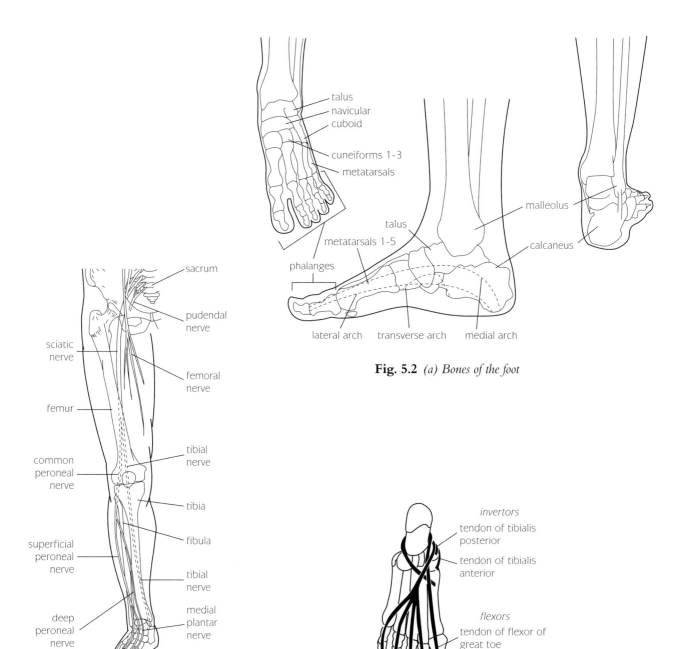

Fig. 5.2 *(a) Bones of the foot*

Fig. 5.2 *(b) Major nerves and tendons of the foot*

Some of the main muscles and ligaments affecting the feet are: the Achilles tendon which originates from the calf muscles and attaches to the calcaneus, the digital flexors on the sole and extensors on the top, the peroneus muscles and the abductors of the legs and feet which can abnormally rotate the feet. The person's posture or the balance of the spinal upper body also affect the balance of weight placed on the feet. Some people present with problems of the foot itself or its biomechanics. When observed, this is referred to a chiropodist, GP or orthopaedic specialist.

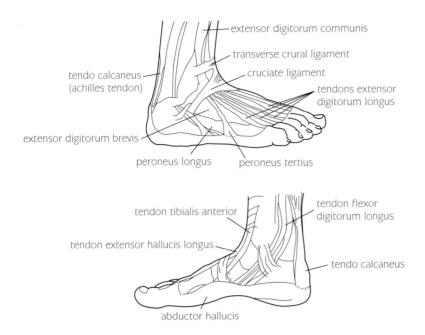

Fig. 5.2 *(c) Muscles and tendons of the foot*

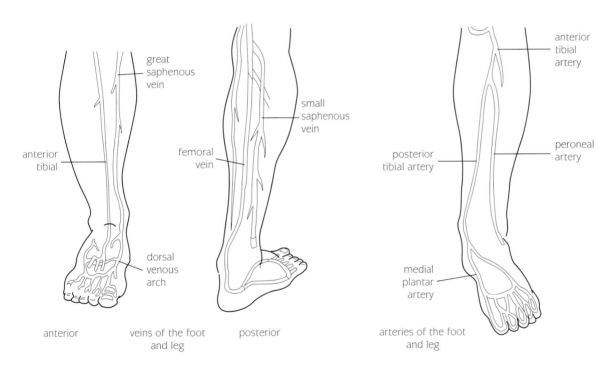

Fig. 5.2 *(d) Circulation of the foot: veins and arteries*

The anatomical feet-whole body correspondences

- Number of bones in the feet: 26; number of vertebrae in the spine: 26.
- Number of curves in the spine and their distribution: 4; number of curves in the spine area of the foot: 4.
- Sizes and proportions of the different body areas on the feet, i.e. head, neck, chest, waistline-abdominal area, and heel correspond to the size and proportion of those areas of the body-whole.
- Head area of the body: toes of the feet, fingers of hands.

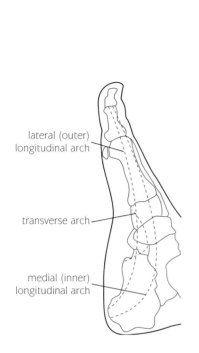

Fig. 5.2 *(e) Arches in the foot*

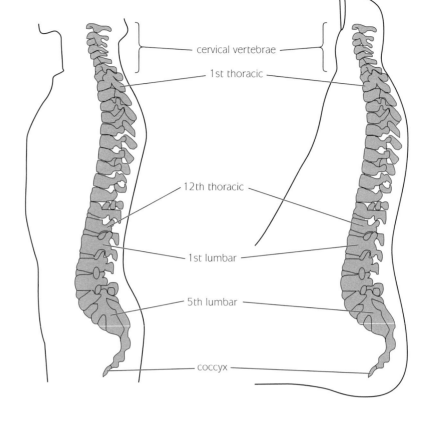

Fig. 5.3 *(a) Reflex area for the spine showing relationship of spine reflex to spine in the body*

- ◆ Chest area of the body: ball of the foot, metatarsal bones.
- ◆ Diaphragm muscle: line of skin change along the lower edge of the ball of the foot.
- ◆ Abdominal area of the body: arch of the sole of the foot.
- ◆ Pelvic area and organs of the body: heel, and the ankle-to-heel area of the foot.
- ◆ Waistline of the body: prominence of the proximal end of the 5th metatarsal bone to the centre point of the medial arch of the foot.
- ◆ Dorsal aspect of foot: the more surface organs and tissues of the body (face, nose, breasts, muscles).
- ◆ Plantar aspect: the more interior organs and tissues (sinus, brain, lungs, heart, colon).
- ◆ Medial aspect: centre of the body.
- ◆ Lateral aspect: outer edge of body.

Cross reflexes

In addition to the above correspondences on the feet themselves, reflexology uses other vital energy correspondences in the body. These are called 'cross reflexes' – anatomical parts of the body which are energetically related; that is, working on any one of them has proved to have an effect on its corresponding part. Cross reflexes are very useful for reinforcing treatment on the foot or for treating a problem when the foot itself is injured, or for helping an injured part of the body by working its cross reflex on the foot. For example if the knee is injured we can give reflexology around the cross reflex, the elbow on the same side of the body. The cross reflexes are:

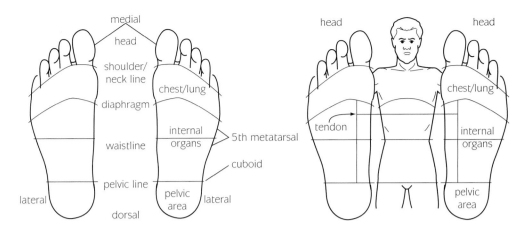

Fig. 5.3 (b) The major areas of the foot divided by the 'landmarks'

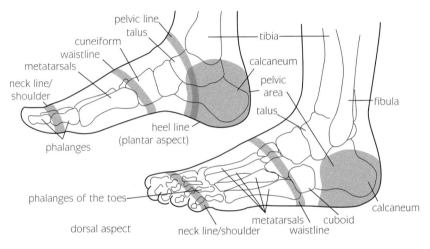

Fig. 5.3 (c) Areas of the foot (shown in colour) superimposed on a diagram of the bones

ankle – wrist
shoulder – hip
elbow – knee
forearm – calf
upper arm – thigh.

REMEMBER
The body is like a hologram; whichever aspect you examine, reveals the nature of the whole.

ACTIVITY
First, examine your own feet and then those of a fellow student or other partner. As you touch the feet, locate the different major areas and features – such as the arches, the metatarsals, the various bones - and simultaneously visualise the parts of the body corresponding to these.

Holistic feet – body correspondences
Vital energy as reflected in the feet
If we see that the vital force is manifested in the differing qualities of energy in the body, these reflect the qualities of earth, water, fire, air and etheric energy. According to Polarity Therapy, these energies are

reflected on the feet in the following areas and any indications in these areas can suggest an imbalance in the flow of that type of energy through the body.

Big toe represents the Etheric element – space through which subtle communication occurs, relates to harmony, clarity.

Second toe represents the Air element – energy as movement, rhythm.

Third toe represents the Fire element – energy as fire and heat, relates to perception, will.

Fourth toe represents the Water element – energy as fluidity, flow, relates to feelings of love, to nurturing, growth.

Fifth toe represents the Earth element – energy as solidity, relates to stability, grounding.

Similarly, the lower area of the foot represents the energy of earth, the lower abdominal area corresponds to that of water, the upper abdominal area to that of fire, the chest area to that of air and the head area to that of ether.

ACTIVITY
Examine your own toes. Feel the temperature and placement of each. Reflect on whether or not this helps you to understand certain aspects of your own life. For example, is your fire energy a little too hot and extroverted, are you perhaps over-working at the moment and needing the balance of cooling water energy and the grounding energy of earth?

GOOD PRACTICE

Gently rubbing the underside of each toe where it joins with the foot and stretching it can help to activate the type of energy flow represented by that toe. For example, if a person needs to have their fire energy strengthened, you can rub the third toe to help stimulate it.

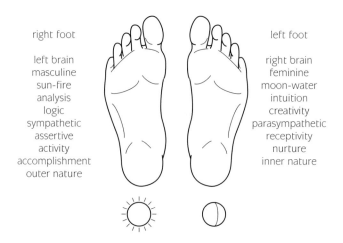

right foot

left brain
masculine
sun-fire
analysis
logic
sympathetic
assertive
activity
accomplishment
outer nature

left foot

right brain
feminine
moon-water
intuition
creativity
parasympathetic
receptivity
nurture
inner nature

Fig. 5.4 *Left-right body-mind correspondences on the feet*

Left-right correspondences

Modern neurology has revealed that each of the brain's hemispheres, the left and the right, is responsible for different types of activity. The left brain is the source of analysis and logic, while right brain faculties are for intuitive and creative mental activities. This agrees with the observations of natural medicine traditions that find energy flows as two qualities through the body, the one symbolised by the sun and male activity, and the other symbolised by the moon and female activity. Because of the cross-over of communications between the brain hemispheres and the body, in the body the right side and hence the right foot is influenced by the left, analytical brain and most reflects 'male' energy and activity. It can indicate how we relate to the masculine aspect of ourselves. The left side and left foot is the 'female side', and relates to the feminine aspect of ourselves.

Whether we are male or female we have each of the two types of energies or potentials within us and in fact the two energies, the two faculties of the hemispheres, are never as separate as the descriptions suggest but are always co-ordinating together. Nevertheless, observing the differences between the left and right feet of our clients may provide useful clues as to the nature or balance of their energy.

> **REMEMBER**
> Each of us has the potential to develop both aspects of ourselves further in positive ways.

The left foot relates to:

- right brain activity
- feminine aspect
- water-moon energies of intuition, receptivity, inner creativity
- para-sympathetic activity, receptivity
- introversion, nurturing
- family relationships, relationships with women and one's feminine side.

Right foot relates to:

- left brain activities
- masculine aspect
- fire-sun energies of will, analysis and logic
- sympathetic nervous system activity
- outer-directed creativity, assertion, extroversion
- worldly relationships, relationships with men and one's masculine side.

In practice, if we find that the left and right feet vary significantly, we can ask ourselves whether, taking into account the person's symptoms, this is perhaps due to an imbalance of left and right brain activity, of masculine and feminine aspects of energy flow. For example, there may be a bunion on one foot and not the other, or one foot may be colder than the other, or have skin symptoms. Such signs are not conclusive in themselves but help us to explore all lines of investigation when trying to understand a person's state of imbalance.

> **GOOD PRACTICE**
>
> When examining your client's feet begin to consider if and how they may reflect a particular right or left brain dominance, as suggested by the speech and appearance of the client. To help balance the hemispheres hold the toes of each foot quietly for a few moments.

Progress Check

1 What are the zone lines?
2 Where are the five elements of energy flow represented on the feet?
3 What are the characteristics of right brain activity?
4 What are the characteristics of left brain activity?
5 What are the cross reflexes?

Using the knowledge

Any significant differences between the appearance or structure of the left and right feet, or the relationship between the structure of the feet and the symptoms the person complains of can indicate areas of imbalance in the person at a physical, emotional or mental level. Such imbalances may lie behind the physical symptoms the person is experiencing. Observe for yourself and use this information, if helpful, to guide your treatments and understanding of your clients. If the person is open to it, such indicators can be used to inform a client about their imbalances and help them to understand themselves better and be more alert to weak areas. It alerts them to their weaknesses but also their strengths.

The landscape of the feet

When working the feet and locating the reflexes, it helps to be familiar with the prominent features and landmarks.

First become oriented to the feet. Each side, top and bottom has a technical name. Notice that when the feet are placed side by side, the imaginary line between them relates to the mid-line of the body. This is the *medial aspect* of each foot, where the spinal reflex is located. The opposite side is the *lateral aspect*. The top of the foot is called the *dorsal aspect* and the bottom, the *plantar aspect*. The toes are the *distal* end of the foot (furthest from the centre of the body), while the ankle and heel are the *proximal* ends. Also the front of the ankle area is *anterior*, or in front of the back of the ankle, the *posterior*.

There are several prominent features or landmarks on the feet. The main ones are:

- the toes, which delineate the head-neck area and its organs
- the ball of the foot, which delineates the thoracic area and its organs
- the change in skin texture under the ball of the foot which locates the diaphragm muscle and divides the thoracic from the abdominal area
- the 5th metatarsal prominence which locates the level of the waistline
- the change of skin at the heel which locates the end of the lower abdominal area and beginning of the pelvic cavity
- the fatty tissue just inside and slightly above the lateral ankle which denotes the bladder area reflex
- the tendon running down the middle of the foot.

ACTIVITY
Palpate your own feet and locate the prominent features and landmarks. Using a washable, coloured pen outline on your feet the landmarks and also the major areas: head, chest, abdomen, pelvis, spine.

REMEMBER
The map represents a conceptual projection of the body onto the foot, based on the correspondences revealed by working on the feet, but in itself is an idealised version of reality, not the reality itself.

The map of foot reflexes
As was pointed out in the introduction, while the majority of reflexes on the feet appear in the same general area on different maps used by reflexologists, there are also several, and quite valid, variations. The map given in this chapter is not intended to be exclusive. However some basic map is needed in a text, so one is provided here. Your teacher may prefer a different one and you will want to follow the map used on your course.

GOOD PRACTICE
Different people have different sized and proportioned feet and indeed even people's inner organs vary slightly in their positions. Learn to 'read' the map in conjunction with what you find on the feet. The map is there to be used to help interpret information, and not to impose an inflexible scheme on a living body.

Progress Check

1 What bones support the arch of the foot?
2 What is the landmark that relates to the waistline?
3 What is the landmark for the pelvic area?
4 Why are there some variations in the maps used by reflexologists?

Conditions of the feet

As a reflexologist is working primarily on the feet of her clients, a basic knowledge of the most common conditions which can affect the feet will be helpful. Conditions on the feet are often related to the general health of the patient or may help explain the origin of certain symptoms the client is experiencing. We know that a disturbance on the foot can disturb the flow of energy through the affected zone and thus create an imbalance and symptoms in the corresponding body part. Always check to see if such disturbance has been affecting other parts of the body in the related reflex or zone.

Being alert to the implications of what is observable on the feet means the reflexologist can better advise her client and when indicated, refer the client to a physician, chiropodist or other appropriate specialist for investigation and treatment.

Some common conditions

Athlete's foot is a contagious fungal infection in which the skin around the toes becomes itchy and red, then white and moist and begins to flake or peel off. Toenails may become yellow and distorted in severe cases. The fungus thrives in warm moist conditions, and is often picked up in swimming pools and changing rooms. Its presence indicates a weakened immune system. Advise clients to wash regularly and dry thoroughly and to expose the feet to air – for example wearing sandals instead of shoes, going bare- or sock-footed – as often as possible. Socks should be of natural materials, not synthetics. Tea tree oil or lemon juice can be healing.

Arthritis is an inflammation of the joints with pain, swelling and heat.

Avulsion is the loss or removal of a toenail due to an accident, injury or corrective surgery, for example, for severe involution.

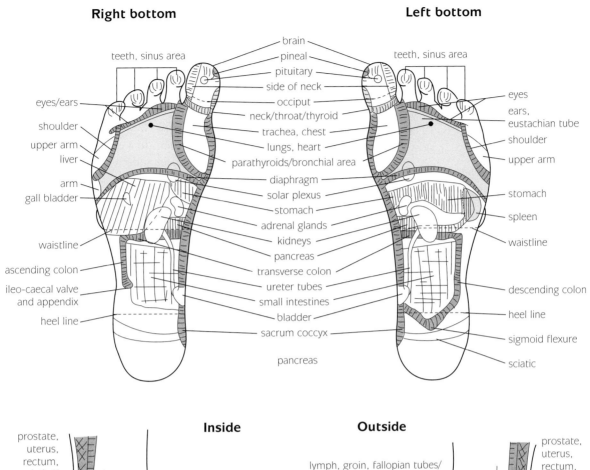

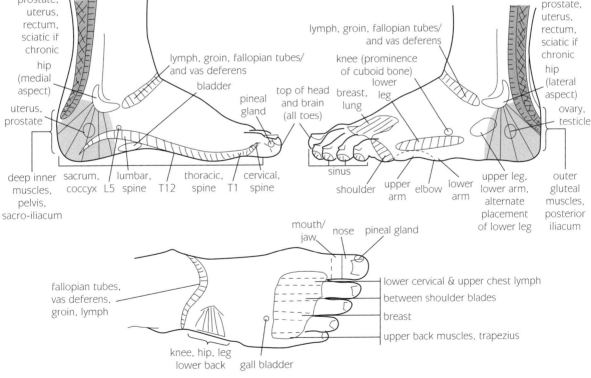

Fig. 5.5 *An example of a map of the feet showing placement of organs. There are variations; for example, some maps show the pituitary at the medial edge of the big toe.*

Bunion, or *hallux valgus*, a weakness at the joint of the big toe and first metatarsal causes the toe to twist inwards towards, over or under the second toe, displacing the joint to the medial side and the big toe laterally. One or both feet may be involved. Pressure, for example from shoes, unbalanced posture or weak arches, may cause or at least worsen the condition, and create callused skin. Inflammations may occur which may eventually lead to degeneration of tissue and osteoarthritis. The person may alter posture to avoid pressure, creating an imbalance in the hips and lower back.

If the condition is very bad, refer the client to a chiropodist; surgery may be indicated. Advice on self-help would include: wearing properly fitting shoes, wearing a toe-pad to help straighten the toe, wearing a protective pad to lessen the discomfort

Bursitis is an inflammation of the *bursa,* or sac, of synovial fluid surrounding and lubricating a joint, for example that of the toe.

Callus and corns form when pressure from constant friction or impact of sufficient force causes an inflammatory reaction within the skin. With pressure, skin cells also reproduce at a faster rate but due to the pressure also become impacted and thicken. If pressure is repeated and focused on one point, a cone of very hard skin is formed called a corn. Ultimate remedy is to remove the cause of pressure, perhaps tight shoes, change of shoes, or imbalanced posture or weight distribution on the feet. Advise the client to visit a chiropodist.

Advice on self-help for callus would include: wearing correctly fitting shoes, using a moulded insole in footwear, wearing felt or foam inserts to lessen discomfort. Refer the client to a chiropodist who may pare away thickened skin or perform surgery if required.

Club nail or ram's horn nail is a disorder in which the nail grows unevenly in a spiral-like manner. The nail usually has a dark discoloration. The commonest cause is a trauma as from a heavy blow or severe stubbing, or from failing to keep the nail short so allowing pressure from footwear which distorts the nail's growth. Sometimes the nail may penetrate the neighbouring toe. Club nail is also when the toenail grows long and over the tip, giving a clubbed appearance. This disorder is often associated with a chronic pulmonary or cardiac condition. Refer to a chiropodist for treatment.

Fallen arches have a variety of causes: weakness or tearing of muscles or ligaments of the feet, excess body weight, prolonged straining from standing or walking, injury, high-heeled shoes, and even malnutrition.

Gout is a very painful inflammation that affects the big toe joint, though it also occurs in knuckles, knees and elbows. Uric acid crystals build up in the joints due to factors such as diet, genetic predisposition, lead poisoning, diuretic drugs, psoriasis; it is also associated with leukaemia. Uric acid, the waste product of protein breakdown, should be excreted in urine, so either too much is being produced because the diet is too high in protein, or kidney function is impaired. Repeated bouts of inflammation degenerate the tissues and deform the joint.

REMEMBER

Listen to the story the individual's feet have to tell. Imbalances lay the foundation for disease.

Hammer toes, a deformity of any of the three middle toes which raises the first phalangeal joint. It may be caused by heredity as in a short first metatarsal segment, which exposes the second and/or third toe to pressure and friction from footwear, or to a bunion; or it may be due to pressure from shoes on the fifth metatarsal which raises the fourth toe. Disease such as arthritis can also deform the toes in this way. The main effect of these abnormalities is that the toes develop painful and persistent corns. Also bursitis, arthritis or painful nail conditions, or ulceration may occur. Referral to a chiropodist is recommended.

Heel spurs are extra growths of bone on the heel caused by the plantar ligaments attaching to the calcaneum becoming inflamed and eroded. If this process is repeated and becomes chronic, new bone is laid down over a period of time and appears as a spur which gives much pain; this sometimes lessens with walking as circulation and drainage improve. The inflammation can be caused by muscle or ligament strain, prolonged standing or ill-fitting footwear. Refer client to a chiropodist for treatment.

High arches, *pes cavus*: the arch is high and therefore more rigid and the toes are pulled backwards and the first metatarsal is pushed down more. Natural shock absorption is reduced and an imbalance is created between the peroneal and tibialis anterior muscles. The cause is unknown, though it can be associated with mild spinal abnormalities or neurological disorders such as polio. Refer client to a chiropodist for treatment.

Ingrown toenails occur when a spur or splinter of the nail or a section of the nail's edge pierces the subcutaneous tissue and if not corrected, continues to grow inward, resulting in inflammation which easily becomes infected. Causes include pressure from footwear, faulty nail cutting, or an abducted gait which increases pressure on the soft tissue at take off. Refer to a chiropodist for treatment.

Nail infections are caused either by bacteria or fungi, which thrive in the warm moist conditions created around the feet by footwear. Older people, diabetics or people with atherosclerosis of the arterial walls are especially prone to these infections. Finding such infections on the nail or foot can alert the reflexologist to the health of the client, who should be advised to check with their doctor or chiropodist.

Osteoporosis is a gradual loss of bone density causing weakening and brittleness of the bone. This occurs naturally with ageing but can occur earlier as a result of such things as prolonged inactivity, calcium deficiency or oral steroid drugs such as those used to treat Cushings Syndrome, asthma and rheumatoid arthritis.

Bone density is maintained by calcium whose metabolism needs calcitonin, produced in the parathyroid glands, and oestrogen; production of these hormones gradually declines with the menopause. Thus the condition is more common in women than men. The reflexologist should handle feet more carefully in this condition and if the client is not already under a doctor's supervision, refer for medical attention.

Verruca is a viral infection of the skin and is infectious. When giving reflexology protect yourself: avoid the infected area or cover it with a plaster, or wear protective gloves.

The feet in diabetic patients

Diabetes has debilitating and degenerative effects on the body which can affect the feet through reduced circulation and reduced nerve supply to muscles and tissues. Poor blood circulation means, for example, the skin of the foot does not heal well even when slightly injured, and infections are also more likely. Skin may become cold, white, dry, hairless. Poor nerve supply – peripheral neuropathy – means the person doesn't feel damages such as tissue breakdown due to calluses. Also loss of sensation moves gradually up the legs over years and can eventually lead to loss of muscle control, toe deformities, pressure problems and impaired sense of balance. Diabetics are advised to examine their feet and hands carefully daily to assess their condition and keep on top of problems.

Progress Check

1   What are two weight-bearing bones in the feet?
2   What is the clinical term for a bunion?
3   How might ill-fitting footwear cause calluses?
4   What is the difference between a corn and a callus?

Key Terms

You need to know what these terms mean. Go back through the chapter or check in the glossary to find out.

- Zones
- Anatomical correspondences
- Cross reflexes
- Distal
- Medial
- Dorsal
- Posterior
- Landmarks
- Major areas
- Left and right brain
- Proximal
- Lateral
- Plantar
- Anterior

PART TWO
REFLEXOLOGY TECHNIQUES

Professional reflexology is based on a sound understanding of anatomy and physiology and of the unique relationship between the feet and hands and the body as a whole. This relationship is itself apparent not only in the many physical reflexes and anatomical correspondences but also through the subtle energy channels found on the feet which affect the organs and systems of the body. Reflexology employs a range of treatment techniques which have originated with pioneers in the field and are continually being developed further by contemporary practitioners. Reflexology lends itself to application in a wide variety of circumstances and for many different types of clients. While usually associated with treatment on the feet, reflexology has always included treatments given to the hands as well and these are as effective, and sometimes more so. Because reflexology aims to restore or enhance the overall health of the whole person, it naturally concerns itself with those aspects of a client's life which have a bearing on health such as diet, exercise and mental and emotional well-being.

REFLEXOLOGY TECHNIQUES

After working through this chapter you will be able to:

- understand that there are variations in reflexology techniques
- use techniques to relax your client before, during and after treatment
- apply the thumb and fingers 'walking' technique
- use effective grips and leverage to vary pressure
- use protective holds to ensure the client's comfort
- understand the importance of good posture and position
- apply the hook-in-back-up technique
- apply rotary or pivoting-on-a-point pressure
- use breathing-on-a-point and light holding techniques to clear blockages
- understand how to vary the basic technique for working specific areas.

Many and varied techniques are used in reflexology. Four or five basic ones are described here because the intention is to provide a basic foundation for your work. However, this is not to promote any one approach as more correct or valuable. Your teacher may well be teaching you other techniques which may differ from or add to the ones discussed in this chapter or may show you some variations. You should aim to master your teacher's techniques. The techniques are described individually in this chapter; a suggested sequence is given in Chapter 7.

Some variations in reflexology techniques are, for example; Linking, developed by Prue Hughes, Light Touch Reflex Action, and the Rwo Shur techniques developed in Taiwan (see Introduction, page xxi). Variations can be seen as natural developments and a sign of the vitality of reflexology, which continues to evolve through the experience of 'what works'. Once qualified, getting together with other reflexologists in your region and exchanging treatments is a good way to experience and learn variations in technique and sequences and to decide which you wish to incorporate.

The aim in mastering any technique is to apply it with sensitivity to the client's response, and to apply it with a smoothness, a flow and a good rhythm while the rest of your body remains as relaxed as possible. These qualities reassure clients and give them confidence in your skills. As with any accomplishment, practice makes perfect, but when practising try not to become too tense or concentrated so that you wear yourself out. Take your time, relax and enjoy your practice.

Relaxation techniques

The relaxation techniques given here are some of the most commonly used and are offered as illustrations of possibilities and as suggestions for you to try. You will want to follow the methods taught by your teacher, and to follow their advice on which techniques to use.

Relaxation techniques are used:

- at the beginning of treatment to relax the client and maximise the effects of the reflexology
- at any time during treatment to maintain relaxation
- at the end of treatment to leave the client in a calm state.

Relaxation techniques, added to your own words and presence, help create the therapeutic environment.

REMEMBER
Before you begin to relax your client, take a moment to centre and relax yourself. Put all thoughts of previous clients or other things out of your mind and be present in the moment.

GOOD PRACTICE

Take care to be extra gentle with older clients and small children when performing these and any reflexology techniques. The bones of elderly people are more brittle and stiff, while children are very sensitive. Both may require a lighter touch.

Greeting the feet

Let your first contact with the feet be light but confident. This is important as it sets the tone for the entire treatment and we wish to enter the client's space with respect. Place both hands beside the feet and take a few breaths to centre yourself. Then place both hands on both feet simultaneously and hold for a few moments. During this contact use your senses to begin to get a feel for the client's state as reflected in the feet. If you have not already done so, observe such things as temperature, blemishes, swelling, dryness or moistness, flexibility, and record your findings.

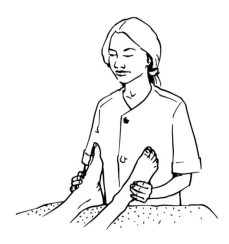

Fig. 6.1 *Light holding of client's feet and centring*

Rhythmic traction

Hold the feet behind the ankles as shown. Stand or sit with your own feet flat and in contact with the floor, your spine relaxed but straight.

Using your bodyweight – not the strength of your arms and hands – gently lean away from the client for about four to five seconds. This traction creates a gentle stretch of the legs which ideally should be felt all the way up through the legs and hips into the upper body. Relax the traction – and your own self – for the same four to five seconds, without loosening your contact.

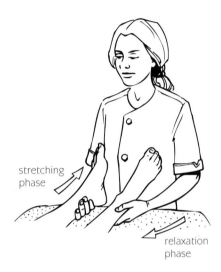

Fig. 6.2 *Rhythmic traction of the feet*

This technique may be omitted for anyone with osteoporosis or the very elderly. Repeat this stretching and relaxing in a gentle, flowing rhythm about five times.

Repeat each of the following techniques on both feet.

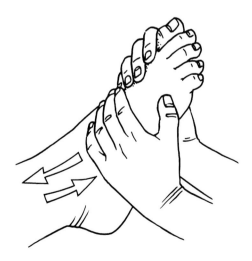

Fig. 6.3 *Effleurage of the foot*

Effleurage

This is simply a gentle massaging of the entire foot with the palms and fingers of the hands. Let your hands be so relaxed that they mould themselves to the contours of the client's foot. Use long, flowing strokes up towards and including the lower leg, and down, round the ankles and back over the soles and toes. Repeat several times.

'Shimmie' vibrations

Place metatarsal edges of one foot between the centres of your palms and while maintaining firm contact, rapidly move your hands from side to side to create a shimmie which loosens the foot. Do not rub the skin between your hands but move the bones beneath the skin by keeping a firm contact.

Repeat this at the ankle area: place the ankle bones between your two palms and rapidly vibrate your hands. If the person is relaxed you should notice the whole foot moving from side to side.

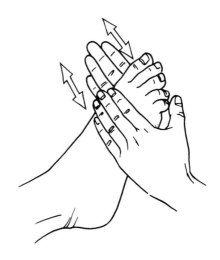

Fig. 6.4 *Shimmie vibrations to the metatarsal area*

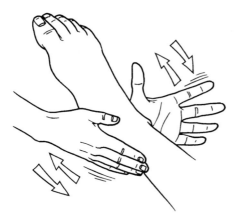

Fig. 6.5 *Shimmie vibrations to the ankles*

If you find the client's foot is a bit stiff, ask them to consciously relax and let go so their foot can move freely. This is a good way of investigating the flexibility of the client's joints.

Once you have mastered this technique, you can begin the shimmie at the metatarsals and then move it down the whole foot to the ankles and back up again, keeping contact all the time.

Rhythmic ankle rotation

Cup the client's heel in the palm of your supporting hand (left hand for client's left foot). Hold the metatarsals with the working hand as shown and rotate laterally four to six times: extend the foot out in a circle then relax your hold slightly to allow the foot to swing back to its natural position.

Add a bit of pressure as you start each rotation and relax your pressure towards the second half of the rotation.

When you have mastered this you can begin to add some traction of the heel by the supporting hand, gently stretching the back of the calf and increasing the flex of the foot.

> **REMEMBER**
> Always work only within the limits of the client's range of movement. Never force the foot into any position.

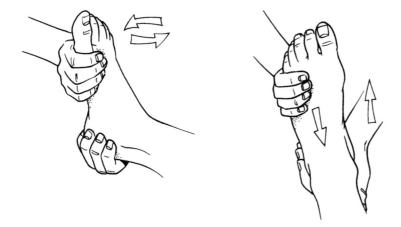

Fig. 6.6 *(a) Ankle rotations (b) Rhythmic ankle stretch and flex*

Rhythmic stretch and flex

Your supporting hand cups the ankle, your working hand holds the metatarsal area. Alternately and rhythmically stretch and flex the top of the foot towards and away from you as you stretch and relax the heel and Achilles tendon area.

Five toes stretch or five element balancing

This technique helps to open the channels of energy flow.

Begin with the big toe, the ether element, and repeat with each of the other toes. Hold the metatarsals with the supporting hand. Grasp the first toe at its base, where it connects with the metatarsals – do not hold the tip of the toe.

1 Gently stretch the toe away from the rest of the foot.
2 Next, still holding the base, gently rotate the toe around the joint with the metatarsal phalange in a side-to-side movement then a full circular movement. Only work within the limits of the client's range of movement.
3 Finally, pull your fingers from the base to the tip of the toe, massaging and stretching the toe as you work.

As you work, be sensitive to how each toe feels. Do you sense any blockage? Congestion? Tension? Stiffness? Excess or deficiency of energy? Too much heat or cold? Note this information for your overall assessment.

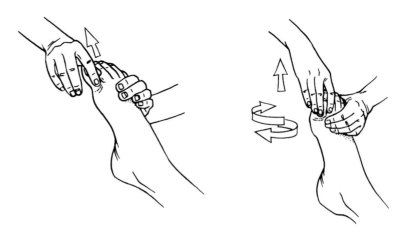

Fig. 6.7 *(a) Five-toe, five element stretch-balancing. (b) Five-toe rotations*

Metatarsal opening

Your supporting hand holds the metatarsals from the dorsal aspect. Form a fist with your working hand and apply the flat of the knuckles against the ball of the foot (plantar metatarsals).

1 Keeping yourself relaxed, gently but firmly lean your body weight towards the client to apply pressure to the ball of the foot while slightly relaxing the hold of the support hand.

   The pressure comes from your body, through your arms and hands, not from any tension of the arm or hand muscles.

2 Relax the body-pressure and, simultaneously, gently compress the metatarsals with your support hand.

3 Repeat this alternation of lateral stretching and closing several times.

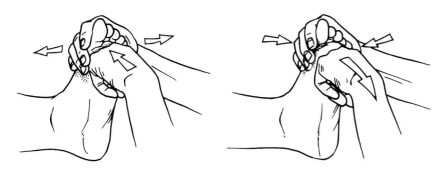

Fig. 6.8 *(a) Metatarsal opening: opening phase, press towards trunk. (b) Metatarsal opening: relaxation phase, gently squeeze metatarsals.*

This movement needs to be done rhythmically and in a flowing manner. It gently opens the metatarsal area of the foot and has a profound effect on the heart and lung reflexes. You may like to visualise the opening of the heart.

> **GOOD PRACTICE**
>
> Giving reflexology involves two hands, the 'working' hand and the supporting/assisting hand. It also involves your whole body, not just the hands and fingers.

Circular frictions

With the finger pads of both hands, make small circles around the ankles and then along the sides of the foot; then up and down the area near the Achilles tendon and the area on the top of the foot at the base of the toes.

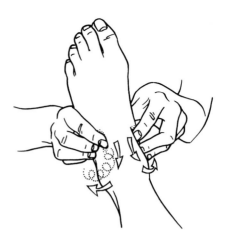

Fig. 6.9 *Circular frictions around ankle*

Criss-cross

With the pads of the thumbs stroke the ball of the foot in a criss-cross manner, thumbs moving back and forth contrary to each other, simultaneously in opposite directions.

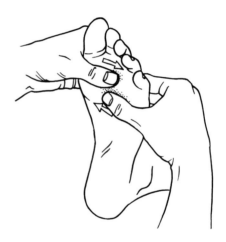

Fig. 6.10 *Criss-cross thumb stroking the sole of the foot*

Knuckle stroking

Make a fist with the working hand and, supporting the foot with the other, stroke the sole with the knuckles vertically up and down and sideways. Be firm but gentle. Pain may be felt especially over the kidney reflexes so be very sensitive in your application. Feet may also be very ticklish with this movement, so you may leave it out.

GOOD PRACTICE

Keep checking yourself for tension which can easily build up as you give treatment. Use your skills of awareness and conscious relaxation to maintain a balanced state within yourself.

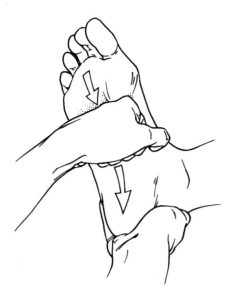

Fig. 6.11 *Knuckle stroking the sole*

Diaphragm–solar plexus release

This is one of the most important techniques in reflexology. It is used whenever the client has experienced a lot of pain as a result of their condition. By releasing tension in the diaphragm muscle, this technique very powerfully helps to release general body tensions, especially the unconscious ones that build up in a body in pain. It also nourishes the nervous system through the solar plexus to aid its recovery.

Place your working thumb on the diaphragm line, zone 1. Hold the metatarsal area with the support hand. With the thumb apply pressure to the first point aiming it to go up and under the bones. Simultaneously lift the metatarsals slightly up, over and on to the thumb.

> **REMEMBER**
> The diaphragm divides the upper and lower parts of the body. Relaxation here improves energy flow between the positive and negative poles of the body.

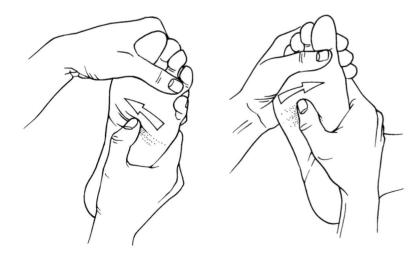

Fig. 6.12 *(a,b) Diaphragm–solar plexus release. Rotate metatarsals onto the thumb placed along the diaphragm line*

Relax all pressure. Move the thumb to the next point along the diaphragm line and repeat the technique. Relax all pressure, move to the next point. Continue, repeating this movement until you have worked along the diaphragm line from medial to lateral; change hands and repeat, moving from lateral to medial.

Make the change of hands effortless and fluid. Keep this a gentle pressure and be sensitive to any tension in this reflex.

GOOD PRACTICE

When you end a relaxing treatment it is a good idea to work the solar plexus reflex (diaphragm line, zone 2) using the breathing-with-pressure technique described on page 98. This induces very deep relaxation and leaves your client in a quiet state at the end of the treatment. Allow the client a few moments in this state before ending the session.

REMEMBER

Each side, top and bottom, of the foot has a technical name. These are explained on page 75.

Spinal twist

First adjust your sitting or standing position to be comfortably facing the medial arch of the foot. Hold the dorsal part of the foot with both hands parallel, thumbs along the sole/plantar aspect, as shown. With the head hand (proximal) remaining still to stabilise that part, use the foot hand (distal) to rotate the foot back and forth laterally.

Start near the ankles and 'twist' in sequential positions as you move toward the toes. Move your hands together only a fraction to the next position to repeat the 'twist'.

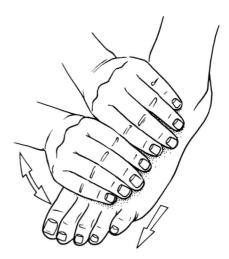

Fig. 6.13 *Spinal twist. Proximal hand stabilises and remains still while distal hand rotates. Move down the foot to the toes, both hands together, twisting gently at each position in the sequence.*

GOOD PRACTICE

Visualisation: as you work, imagine the spine as a golden cord and that you are holding each vertebra in turn and gently twisting it back and forth to loosen the muscles and release tension. Keep your movements rhythmic and flowing.

Reflexology pressure techniques

After years of trial and error, Eunice Ingham settled on a special compression touch technique as the most effective way of giving treatment. Many reflexologists use this technique or variations of it, and many reflexologists have developed other techniques. The technique is often called thumb and finger 'walking' – words which try to capture its distinct nature of slow, purposeful and rhythmic movements across the foot.

The importance of rhythm

It is little noticed that this very simple technique combines a pressure phase with a relaxed phase, creating a rhythmic alternation of pressure with non-pressure which has profound effects on the body. It acts on the para-sympathetic nervous system, which is especially sensitive to stimulation by deliberate rhythmically applied pressures. This is the aspect of the autonomic system which is responsible for rest and repair, for recovery of energy.

No matter which technique is used, a natural, smooth flow or rhythmic pressure should be the aim.

Thumb and finger walking technique

The aims of the technique:

- the foot can be covered effectively and efficiently without missing any reflex points
- each part of the foot can be explored sensitively to assess any imbalances in the body.

Visualisation

Think of your thumb and fingers as exploring or searching the foot, seeking out, probing – but in a highly sensitive way – the foot to detect imbalances, irritations, blockages to the client's health. Try to put your mind, your conscious awareness into the tip of your thumb or finger so that your hands, fingers and thumbs experience and register what you are sensing there. Become aware of each nuance of tension in the person's foot, of any irregularities in the tissues beneath the surface such as congestion, grittiness, lumpiness, heat, cold.

The movement is characterised by:

- a phase of pressure onto a specific point followed by a brief but definite phase of relaxation of the pressure without losing contact with the skin. There is pressure, then briefly no pressure

- pressure is given at minute intervals, but without skipping over any area of skin and hence treating each reflex point
- an on-going forward movement along the skin. Forward here means toward the next point of skin away from the thumb or finger tip
- sensitively watching the client's face to note how they are reacting to the pressure so that it may be adjusted as needed.

Method

1 Flex the first joint of the thumb or finger and apply precise, pin-point pressure, deeply or lightly as needed, slightly to the medial edge of the digit and slightly proximal to the tip. Pressure is directly down into the body tissues.

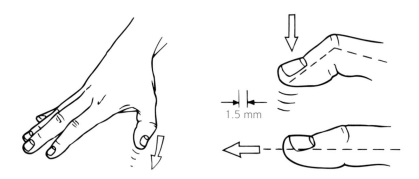

Fig. 6.14 *(a) Thumb walking technique. Flex thumb at first joint and move forward in very small stages (1.5 mm). Practise until you can move incrementally while keeping shoulders and arm relaxed. (b) Thumb walking showing pressure phase – directed down and in – and relaxation phase*

2 Apply pressure not at right angles to the point but at about a 45° angle. Right angle pressure is sometimes used in specific ways but not during the forward movement.
3 Use mainly the medial edge of the thumb close to but not on the tip.
4 Relax the pressure but do not lose contact with the skin.
5 Do not consciously move the thumb or finger forward. Forward movement automatically occurs without effort, simply by the nature of the pressure-relaxation movement.
6 Allow the touch to originate in the centre of the body and come up through the caring heart, down the arms and hands into the thumb or finger.

REMEMBER

Be sensitive at all times. Watch the person's face and eyes. Sense with your hands when pressure is too firm or uncomfortable. Adjust your pressure to the client's tolerance.

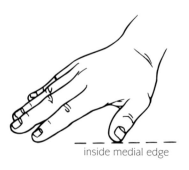

inside medial edge

Fig. 6.15 *Thumb walking practice using inside medial edge*

Uses

This technique is used to cover the majority of the foot reflexes. It is an efficient way to contact the greatest number of reflexes in a reasonable amount of time.

ACTIVITY

First practise on yourself. Sit in a chair and practise the thumb walking on your thigh, starting near the body and moving towards the knee. Work down in rows. Feel for yourself the 'pressure/no pressure' of the movement. Practise maintaining contact with the skin on the relaxation phase. Practise allowing the forward movement to happen by itself without making it happen. Experiment with different pressures and notice how each feels and makes you feel. Repeat using the index and third fingers.

Once you have begun to master the technique, practise it on your own feet. Sit with one foot across the opposite knee and apply the technique along the sole of your foot. Repeat on other parts of the foot that can be reached comfortably. Use the thumbs and fingers of each hand.

Now practise the movement on a partner or fellow student. Experiment with different pressures and give each other feedback as to how they feel and make the receiver feel.

Leverage

Once you have mastered the thumb walking technique, learn to use leverage to your advantage. This has the advantage of increasing penetration without increasing any effort on the part of the working thumb.

To use leverage, as you apply pressure with the working thumb, use the other fingers of the working hand which are wrapped around the foot to bring the foot towards or onto the thumb. You 'pull' the foot onto your thumb.

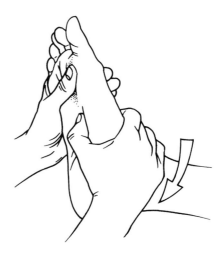

Fig. 6.16 *Leverage: pulling with fingers, palm and wrist in and down to pull the foot onto the thumb*

Support and protection

When giving treatment, the non-working hand is used to support the foot, and to place and maintain it in the most advantageous position for application of pressure to different reflexes. This is important to gain better access to the reflex points and enhance penetration of the touch.

Support holds

When working the foot, use the support hold as follows:

- with the supporting hand, gently tip the toe-metatarsal area of the foot back to expose the plantar aspect to the working hand
- when you are working the spine, the support hand holds the foot so the working thumb and finger can move efficiently and effectively
- when working the pelvic area, use the supporting hand to hold the foot upright to expose the area to the working hand. Alternatively, tilt the foot slightly to expose the area.

Protection hold

Some parts of the feet are particularly sensitive and a hold is needed which protects the client from being pinched between your thumb and

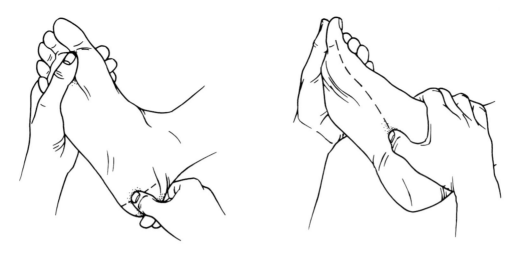

Fig. 6.17 *(a,b) Support holds: left hand supports and positions the foot*

fingers. This is especially true of the toe area and the lymphatic area near the toes, where it is easy for the thumb and fingers to become like pincers around the toes.

To prevent this, when working on the toes, on the pituitary, pineal, lymph or other vulnerable part with the thumb, always use the protection hold.

Place the fingers of your supporting hand between the thumb and fingers of the working hand as shown.

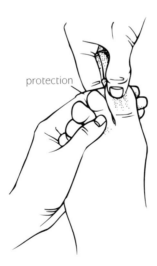

protection

Fig. 6.18 *Protection hold: fingers of support hand betweeen the thumb and fingers of the working hand*

Working a specific reflex point

'Working' a point or reflex means application of reflexology techniques, such as thumb-finger walking, or light holding to a particular reflex which has been found to be tender, congested or tense, or which can help improve the condition the client is experiencing.

Walking technique

When you find a tender or congested area, work over it several times with the thumb-walking technique. Work from different angles and use each hand: work horizontally, vertically and diagonally over the point. After a few moments of work, ask your client if the tenderness lessens at all as you work the reflex. For sensations of tension or congestion, ask yourself if you feel any change in the tissues beneath your fingers. Record whether it changes or remains the same. Next leave the point, moving on to work other reflexes but come back to it at the end of the treatment and work it again to see if there has been any change or if it has remained the same.

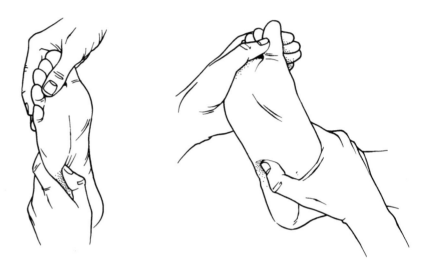

Fig. 6.19 *(a) Working a reflex from different angles, using both hands*

Breathing-with-pressure

When reflexes are particularly congested or painful, this technique serves two purposes. First, it can help to clear the blockages more quickly and secondly, it prevents the client from tensing against the pressure you apply.

An important bonus is that it engages the client in her own process of self-healing. You and the client work together to free the body from the things that are interfering with its harmony and balance.

Place your working thumb or finger on the tender reflex, with only a light pressure at first, just enough to make contact with the tenderness. Explain to your client that you would like her to take five deep but gentle, abdominal breaths. You would like her to breathe deeper into abdomen and to make the exhalation a little longer.

Ask her, as she exhales, to imagine that she is breathing into and through the tender reflex on the foot and to feel that the *out* breath is carrying away with it any congestion, tension or pain in the reflex. Ask her to relax into the breathing, letting her body become loose and soft. It helps if you synchronise your breathing with the client's. Make your out breath a little audible by slightly closing off the back of the throat.

Repeat this with the next four breaths. With each out breath gradually increase the pressure a little more on the reflex point. At the end of five breaths, ask your client to breath normally while you maintain a light contact with the reflex point for a few moments more.

Later in the treatment return to the reflex to check if it is still as tender as it originally was. Any lessening of tenderness means the reflex and the corresponding area of the body have cleared somewhat. Often you can feel the change in the tissues beneath your fingers, or the point warming up, or the tension releasing at that reflex – these also signify a shift towards clearing in the body part. Repeat this as needed.

GOOD PRACTICE

Maintain eye contact and verbal communication throughout the treatment – unless the client wishes to close her eyes and be quiet. Keep checking the client's responses, inviting feedback to engage them in the treatment process. Be open to what your fingers are telling you about the client's state.

Light holding pressure

As an alternative to working over a tender or congested reflex point with repeated passes of the thumb-walking technique, try this light holding technique. You may be impatient with it at first – perhaps feeling that you are not doing anything – but with practice you will become more comfortable with it.

Simply place your thumb or finger on the point with light but confident contact. Leave the thumb there while you practise breathing awareness for about one to two minutes – wait with patience. Usually you will feel a shift in the point; often it warms up or the congestion lessens slightly. This is a sign that the energy has increased through the point – and thus to the corresponding body part – and the area has improved. Try thumb walking over the point again now to test if it is still as tender or tense as it originally was.

Hook-in-back-up technique

This technique is used by some schools on reflex points which are quite small, deep and/or specific. For example, among others:

◆ pituitary
◆ pineal
◆ ileo-caecal valve
◆ appendix
◆ sigmoid colon.

Flex the thumb and place it almost vertically to the point, approaching a 90° angle. Next press, directing pressure first IN or DOWN into the foot (hook-in phase). Then, maintaining that pressure, pull the thumb back toward the centre of the hand, with a dragging effect to the tissues under the skin (back-up phase).

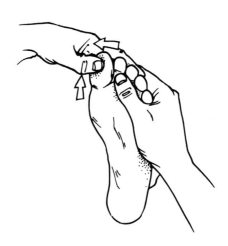

Fig. 6.20 *Hook-in-back-up technique on the pituitary*

Pivot-on-a-point technique

This technique is used primarily to work the diaphragm-solar plexus area and the adrenal glands, but may be used wherever it is needed and practicable.

Place the flexed thumb on the reflex point. Now with the supporting hand, bring the foot onto the thumb. Maintain pressure while rotating the foot slightly on the thumb which acts as the pivot point.

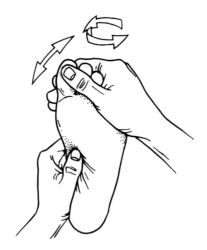

Fig. 6.21 *Pivot-on-a-point technique on the adrenal glands*

Support technique for working the toes

When working the toes, use the thumb and fingers of the supporting hand to elongate and stabilise the toe, maximising the surface area to the working thumb and finger. This support enables you to work 'down' the toe from tip to metatarsal joint as well as 'up'.

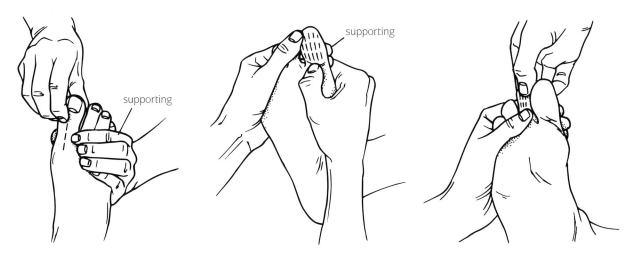

Fig. 6.22 *(a,b,c) Support technique for working the toes: index and thumb stabilise the toe while the working hand works up or down*

GOOD PRACTICE

Always use a protecting hold when working the toes (page 96).

Support technique for working the upper lymph reflex area

Make a loose fist with the supporting hand and place the knuckles flat against the ball of the foot. Place the thumb of the working hand inside the fist, leaving the index or third finger free to work the reflexes. Start at the base of the first toe and work toward the ankle (proximal direction) in the natural groove between the metatarsal bones. Simultaneously exert gentle pressure against the ball to open the metatarsal area. Work from medial to lateral in each groove, then change hand positions fluidly and return, working lateral to medial.

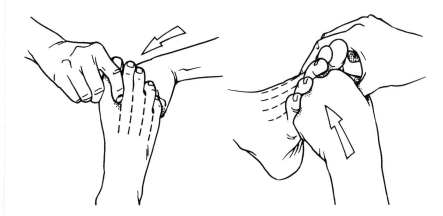

Fig. 6.23 *(a,b) Support technique for working the neck-chest lymphatic reflexes*

Working the eye-ear reflexes

The supporting hand holds the metatarsal area with the thumb pulling the skin down slightly to expose the eye-ear reflexes. Using the index or third finger of the working hand, work across the area from lateral to medial. Exchange hands fluidly and make a return journey with the other hand working the reflexes medial to lateral.

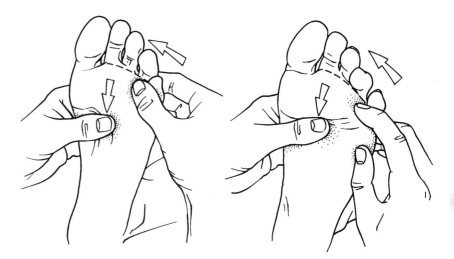

Fig. 6.24 *(a,b) Working the ear-eye reflexes, with either thumb or finger*

For more specific work, place the finger or thumb pad on a point along the reflex and give repeated alternating pressure. Use the breathing technique to release the area. Repeat as needed at individual points along this reflex area.

Working the bladder-kidney reflexes

With the supporting hand hold the client's foot and gently tilt it laterally, exposing the bladder reflex. Place the thumb of the working hand on the bladder reflex and, directing the movement from ankle to toes, use the walking technique to work over the reflex area in sections or 'strips' until you cover the entire reflex. Repeat with the other hand working 'down' the reflex from toes towards the ankle.

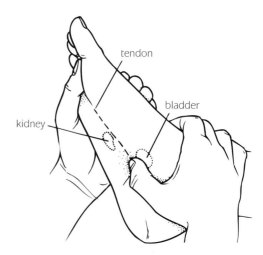

Fig. 6.25 *Working the bladder to kidney reflexes*

Place the thumb of the working hand on the bladder reflex and use the walking technique to work from the bladder up the ureter reflex to the kidney reflex area. When you reach the kidney reflex, work it in strips or sections as described above for the bladder reflex.

REMEMBER
The kidney and bladder reflex may be quite tender on many people. Observe carefully and adjust your pressure accordingly.

Working the chronic uterus-prostate-rectum area
The supporting hand holds the foot so it is slightly flexed to expose the reflex area next to the Achilles tendon. Working with the index or third finger, work up the reflex area from heel to calf.

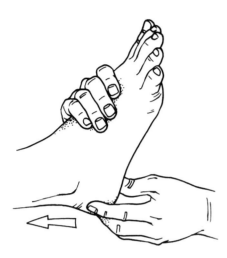

Fig. 6.26 *Working the chronic uterus–prostate–rectum area*

Alternatively, place the working hand on the lower leg and, using the thumb, work down the reflex from calf to heel. Repeat the movements several times to work the area thoroughly.

Working the uterus-prostate reflex
The working hand holds the heel of the foot with the third finger on the uterus-prostate reflex point. The supporting hand holds the foot at the metatarsals and rotates the foot as pressure is applied by the finger to the point.

Working the ovaries-testes reflexes
Hold the heel in the palm of the working hand, with the third finger on the reflex point. Apply gentle but firm pressure directly into the point, then relax. Repeat this several times.

REMEMBER
Tenderness in this area does not always mean imbalance. It could be that there has been an operation here, or, for women, that the period is just about to start, or ovulation occur.

GOOD PRACTICE

When either of these two reflexes is particularly tender, use the light holding pressure (page 99) on both points simultaneously for a few minutes.

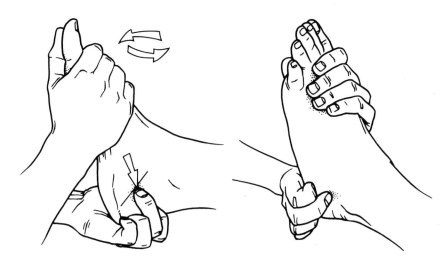

Fig. 6.27 *(a) Working the uterus–prostate area, rotation technique (b)Working the ovary-testes area, pressure technique*

Working the pelvic area

Work generally over the pelvic area as follows; the area may be worked simultaneously with both hands or one side at a time.

Simultaneous working: support and slightly flex the foot with the thumb placed on the ball of the foot. Place the working fingers at the edge of the foot and work, using the walking technique, up toward the ankle. Work in sections starting at the toe end and moving to the Achilles tendon. Work diagonally towards the ankle as shown.

Single-side working: the support hand gently tilts the foot to expose the area. Using either the thumb or finger(s), work the area, in sections, as below. Work from the edge of foot to ankle, from ankle to edge and horizontally across the area.

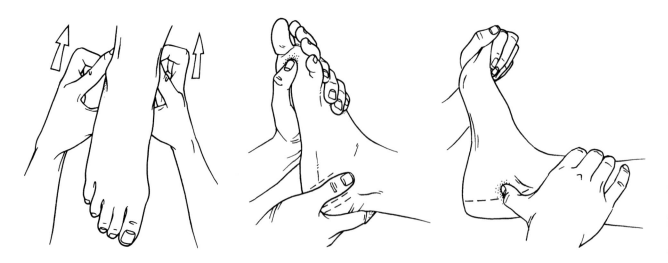

Fig. 6.28 *(a) Working the pelvic area, both sides simultaneously. (b,c) Working the pelvic area, each side separately*

Working the lower lymph reflexes

The supporting hand holds the foot in flexion as for working the pelvic area. Place the index fingers of each hand at the lower part of the reflex as shown and work in the natural groove below the malleolus (ankle) bone up and around towards the top and centre of the area.

As you near the top, stop working with one hand and stabilise the skin while the other index finger continues to the centre. Then repeat this with the other hand.

You can also work this reflex area by using fingers to work down over the area from the toe end towards the body. You can work it by using the thumb, one side at a time to work from the malleolus to the top of the foot.

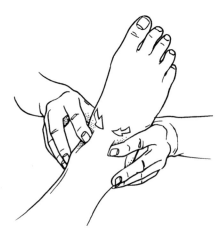

Fig. 6.29 *Working lower lymph/fallopian tube, vas deferens area*

Working the sciatic reflex

The supporting hand holds the foot and gently flexes it to expose the area. Place the thumb of the working hand on the edge of the foot at the middle of the heel area, zone 1. Stabilise the foot with the four remaining fingers. Work across the sciatic reflex with the thumb from medial to lateral several times. Exchange hands fluidly and repeat from lateral to medial.

Working the sciatic loop

Begin the movement at a point just above the point of the ankle and work down to the middle of the heel line, work across the sciatic line. Exchange hands and repeat with the other hand.

Working the large intestine-colon reflex

The supporting hand gently flexes the foot to expose the area. Place the thumb of the working hand on the heel line, zone 1. Work down towards the middle of the heel area at a 45° angle. Repeat several times. From the middle of the heel area, pivot the thumb and work towards zone 1 at a 45° angle, finishing at the heel line, zone 5.

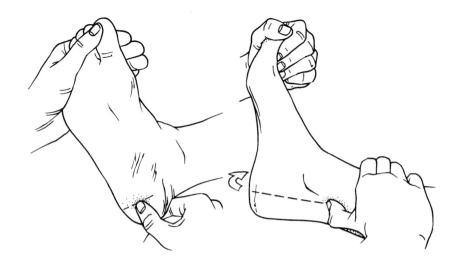

Fig. 6.30 *(a) Working the sciatic reflex under the heel (b) Working the sciatic reflex, from the chronic area*

Also work the sigmoid reflex using the hook-in-back-up technique described above. Having worked the sigmoid colon, place the working hand at zone 5, on the heel line and work up the lower bowel reflex to the transverse colon, pivoting the thumb at the waistline. Work horizontally across the foot to zone 1. Repeat several times as needed.

Pick up the reflex on the right foot, waistline, zone 1. Work horizontally across the transverse colon reflex. Repeat several times as needed.

Work the ascending colon using the left hand, while the right hand supports and flexes the foot gently. Work up the ascending colon to the hepatic flexure reflex area.

REMEMBER

Identify the heel line by the change in skin texture.

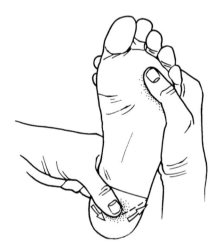

Fig. 6.31 *Working the sigmoid-rectum colon area reflex*

GOOD PRACTICE

If working on skin that is too moist or sticky for your hands, you may wish to lubricate with cornflour.

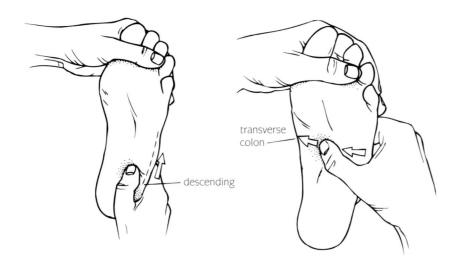

Fig. 6.32 *(a,b) Working up the descending colon, horizontally across the transverse colon. Left foot*

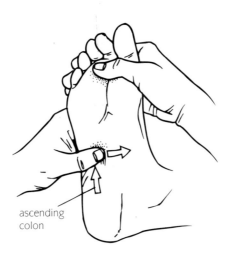

Fig. 6.33 *Working the transverse colon horizontally on the right foot*

Shoulder-arm-elbow reflex

The supporting hand positions and stabilises the foot while the index finger or thumb works up the reflex from the waistline, changing hands to work down. Also work into and around the joint of the fifth metatarsal from the dorsal, plantar and medial aspect, as you gently traction the little toe to create space.

Working reflexes in the chest, upper and lower abdomen

It is convenient to divide the area into three sections:

- ◆ diaphragm line to neck line for lungs, oesophagus, thyroid helper reflexes
- ◆ waistline to diaphragm line for stomach, pancreas, liver, spleen reflexes
- ◆ heel line to waistline for small intestine reflexes.

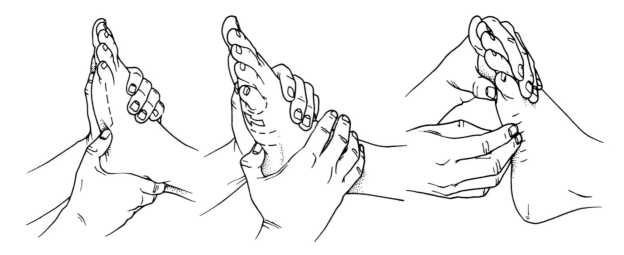

Fig. 6.34 *(a,b,c) Working the shoulder–arm–elbow reflex*

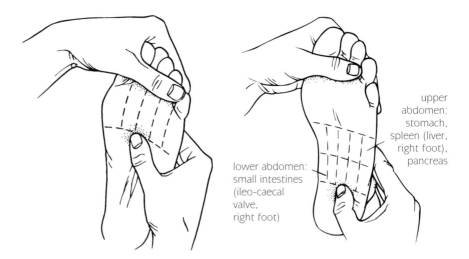

lower abdomen:
small intestines
(ileo-caecal
valve,
right foot)

upper
abdomen:
stomach,
spleen (liver,
right foot),
pancreas

Fig. 6.35 *(a) Working the plantar chest reflex for oesophagus, bronchioles, thyroid helper. (b) Working the upper abdomen reflexes for stomach, pancreas, liver and spleen. Working lower abdomen reflexes for small/large intestine*

Each section may be worked in several ways:

- ◗ work vertically up each zone in each section, working with the thumb of one hand medially to laterally, and changing hands fluidly, working back laterally to medially. Repeat as needed
- ◗ work across the area diagonally in strips
- ◗ work across the area in horizontal strips
- ◗ work specific organ or tender/congested reflexes in detail by working onto them from many different angles; by applying breathing-with-pressure techniques; by working with a rotary motion into a specific tender or congested area.

Working the thyroid and parathyroid glands reflex
On some charts this reflex is located around the base of the big toe; other charts show it in other positions. The parathyroid glands reflex on some charts is the same as that for the thyroid gland; on others it has a separate location.

To work the thyroid/parathyroid, the supporting hand positions and stabilises the foot. Using either the thumb and index fingers or both, work across the reflex from medial to lateral. Work from one direction with one hand and from the opposite with the other. Work it from below up in sections.

Some charts also show a 'helper' thyroid reflex located in the chest area between the first and fifth metatarsal bones, from waistline to neck line. This reflex has also been found to help in thyroid conditions. To work this, start on the waistline with the thumb and work up to the thyroid reflex. Change hands and repeat with the other thumb.

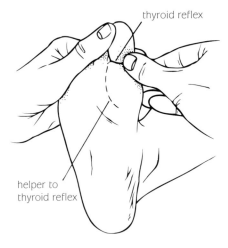

thyroid reflex

helper to
thyroid reflex

Fig. 6.36 *Working the thyroid reflex*

Working the head-sinus reflexes
Method one
The supporting hand stabilises and protects the toe as described on page 96. Raise your arm slightly so as to be able to start the movement from the tip of the toe. Beginning in the middle, work down the medial area as far as possible, pick up your thumb and work down the lateral area. If the toe is large, you may work down a further section. Repeat on the four remaining toes. Change hands and work in the same way from lateral to medial, this time starting again with the middle section and repeating on the medial sections of the toes.

Method two
The supporting hand stabilises and protects. With the working thumb, begin at the base of the toe and work vertically up, again sectioning the toe off into strips and working up each strip.

Other techniques:

- work up and down the sides of the toes to work the neck area
- work around the front of the toe horizontally in sections using the finger to work the face reflexes. Work from both lateral and medial directions
- using the tip of the index or third finger, roll firmly over the tip of the toes to stimulate the brain reflexes.

Working the spinal reflexes
First stage

The supporting hand holds the metatarsal area and tilts the foot gently outwards, exposing the area. Place the heel in the fingers of the working hand and the thumb on the starting point, the coccyx reflex. Work up the spine as far as you comfortably can before your thumb stretches too far from your fingers – about the 5th lumbar reflex. Next, leaving the thumb in contact, release your fingers and swivel them round to hold the foot from the dorsal aspect, pivoting around the thumb. Now continue to work up the spine to the last cervical reflex.

Shift your fingers and thumb as you move up, as needed.

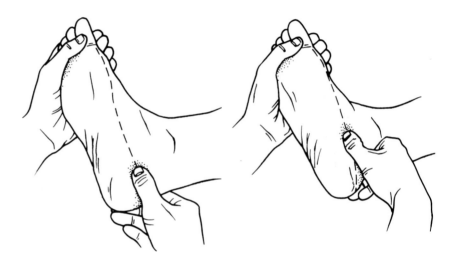

Fig. 6.37 *(a,b) Working the spinal reflex, first stage*

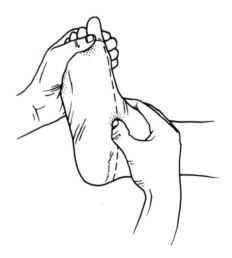

Fig. 6.37 *(c) Working the spinal reflex, first stage*

Second stage

Change hands. Place the back of the supporting hand along the sole of the foot, stabilising and supporting. The working thumb starts at the top of the spinal reflex, approximately at the base of the big toe nail. Stabilise the thumb by using the four fingers on the dorsal aspect.

Work down the spine to the coccyx.

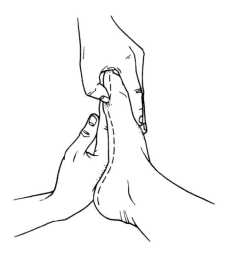

Fig. 6.38 *Working the spine from neck down to coccyx with support hand and wrist stabilising the foot*

Third stage

To work specific areas of the spine, apply the above techniques in detail. In addition, use the thumb or index and third fingers to work horizontally across the spinal reflex points. Pivot-on-a point techniques can also be used for specific vertebrae.

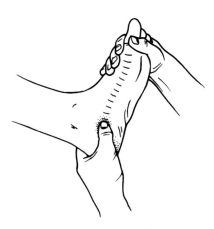

Fig. 6.39 *Working specific areas of the spine horizontally*

> **REMEMBER**
> The spine is more than just a thin line of reflexes. It is quite wide and corresponds not only to the vertebrae but also to the cartilage (discs), nerves and muscles attaching to the spine.

Tips for specific points:

- the 5th lumbar may be worked with pivoting-on-the-thumb technique

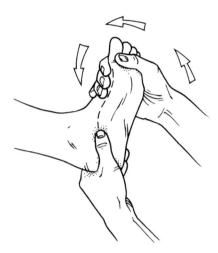

Fig. 6.40 *Working the 5th lumbar area*

- the neck area may be worked in detail using the index finger as well as the thumb

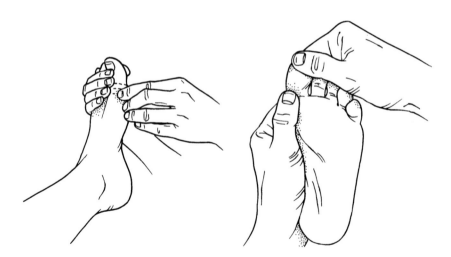

Fig. 6.41 *Working the neck area*   **Fig. 6.42** *Working the occiput area*

- the occiput of the cranium may be worked using individual thumb pressures, direct or rotary, along the base of the pad of the big toe.

Working the knee-hip-leg reflex
The supporting hand stabilises and positions the foot by slightly tilting it inwards. Start with the thumb or index and third fingers at the bony prominence of the navicular bone. Work down towards the lateral edge of the foot. Divide the area into sections and work down each.

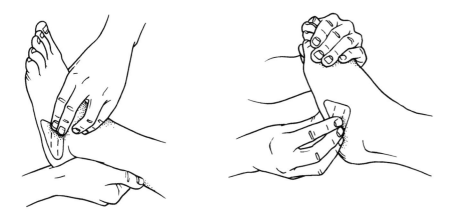

Fig. 6.43 *(a,b) Working the knee–hip–leg reflex*

Change hands and work up from the lateral edge of the foot towards the navicular prominence, in sections as needed.

Working the hip reflex
The supporting hand slightly flexes and stabilises the foot. Work in one or more of the following ways.

Method one
Use the index and/or third fingers to work from the proximal end beneath and around the malleolus.

Method two
Use the thumb or fingers to work from distal beneath and around the side of the malleolus.

Method three
Use the thumb or fingers to work up to and onto the hip reflex in sections from the lower edge of the foot, lateral and medial.

REMEMBER
The lateral hip reflex corresponds to the lateral area of the hip joint and the medial to the medial area of the hip joint. Similarly, the more anterior of the reflex corresponds to the anterior hip area while the posterior reflex corresponds to the more posterior.

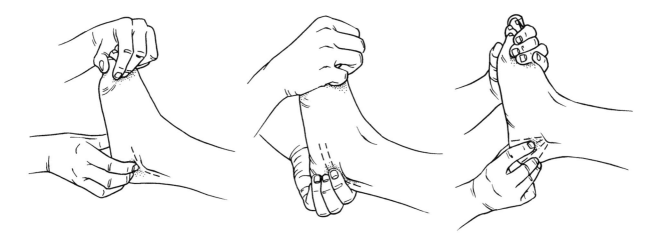

Fig. 6.44 *(a,b,c) Working the hip reflex, under the ankle, methods 1,2 and 3*

When working the hip reflexes also work the pelvic area well for the gluteal and deeper muscles of the buttocks and work the entire spine to help align the pelvis correctly.

ACTIVITY

Practise each of the above techniques on your own feet first as far as possible. Note how you respond in your health journal. Try different pressures, e.g. very light to quite deep and penetrating, noticing the differences in the way each makes you feel.

Practise each of the above techniques on a partner. Try out different pressures. Ask your partner to give you feedback on how working the reflex makes them feel.

Key Terms

You need to know what these terms mean. Go back through the chapter or check in the glossary to find out.

- Distal
- Plantar
- Lateral
- Thumb walking
- Posterior
- Breathing-with-pressure
- Thyroid helper
- Proximal
- Dorsal
- Medial
- Anterior
- Hook-in-back-up
- Sciatic loop

THE TREATMENT SEQUENCE AND GIVING A WHOLE FOOT TREATMENT

7

After working through this chapter you will be able to:

♦ prepare a client for a reflexology treatment

♦ give reflexology treatment to the whole of both feet

♦ understand the importance of maintaining communication with the client and engage her in the process of the treatment

♦ adapt the treatment to varying circumstances and individual needs of clients

♦ understand the location of reflexes for specific systems of the body.

The treatment sequence given in this chapter is a good basic one to follow. It is not the only one possible and many reflexologists use a different sequence. It is given to illustrate how the techniques described in Chapter 6 may be put together to form a coherent treatment and can perhaps also form the basis for discussion about different styles. Your teacher may well teach you another sequence and this is what you will want to learn and follow.

It is a good idea to learn a basic sequence and become proficient at it before varying and adapting it further. The aim in the sequence is to stimulate the most important reflexes within a 45- to 50-minute treatment session, while allowing time to also work specific reflexes relevant to the client's condition. This way the client receives a whole foot treatment at each visit, while also receiving treatment on the symptoms and causes of her ailments.

Preparing for the treatment

After taking the client's case history, ask her to lie or sit in a comfortable position and see to her comfort with towels and supporting cushions as needed. Some practitioners like to ask the client to indicate verbally if she senses tenderness or other sensation at a reflex; and they might prompt with the occasional question, such as 'How does this reflex feel to you?' In addition, of course, they watch the client's face and body for indications and pay attention to what their own touch tells them. Other therapists prefer to rely on non-verbal indicators and intuition.

Some general suggestions about treatment

♦ Different reflexologists and teachers have evolved different routines that work well for them. For example, many reflexologists start with the left foot, work the whole foot, then proceed to the right foot. They then return to work reflexes of specific systems, tissues and organs on both feet as needed. Others prefer to work both feet together by systems, for example the lymph system on both feet, then the digestive system, and so on. Sometimes the sequence is to work up each of the five zones on the soles of the feet and then work specific reflexes. This is especially useful if time is limited. Once you have learned a basic sequence, as you gain experience, you can adapt and modify the sequence as you think consistent with good results.

♦ Always begin with relaxation techniques to both feet. Cover the foot not being worked on with a towel for warmth.

♦ Work each general area thoroughly in the way you have been taught, for example, first with one hand medial to lateral and then the other lateral to medial, working in sections vertically, horizontally or diagonally as desired.

♦ Work specific reflexes inside general areas as you go. For example, hook-in-back-up on the ileo-caecal reflex in the abdomen; stomach reflexes in the abdomen; or light holding touch on the neck reflexes. An alternative method is to work the whole foot and then come back to give attention to specific reflexes.

♦ Use one or more relaxation techniques after working a tender point.

♦ Use relaxation techniques at intervals during treatment to relax the client and yourself.

♦ Ensure contact is warm, confident and reassuring.

♦ Keep a flow and rhythm of movement as you change hands or feet.

♦ See to the client's comfort at all times.

♦ Observe the client's face throughout and confirm her responses verbally, if necessary.

♦ Start with moderate pressure and check with the client as you proceed, asking for feedback. Alter pressure as necessary. Lightest pressure, and light holding can also be used throughout.

♦ Record your findings as you work.

♦ End the treatment with solar plexus breathing-with-pressure. Hold the feet passively for a few moments to help balance the body. Allow the client to relax a few minutes in the stillness to absorb the experience, before ending the session.

♦ Remind the client what to expect after treatment and how to care for herself.

♦ If appropriate, teach the client to work specific reflexes herself in the interval before the next treatment.

 Progress Check

1 Why is it important that the client is well informed about the nature of reflexology and the importance of her participation in the treatment?

2 What two means other than the client's verbal communication, tell you how the client is responding to the reflex stimulations?

3 Why is it a good idea to use relaxation techniques throughout the treatment, not just at the beginning or end?

4 Why is it important to keep a rhythmic flow of movements over the feet?

A basic sequence

Refer to Chapter 6 for details of how to work the reflexes if needed.

1   Make contact with the feet, and hold them passively for a few moments while you relax yourself and centre in.

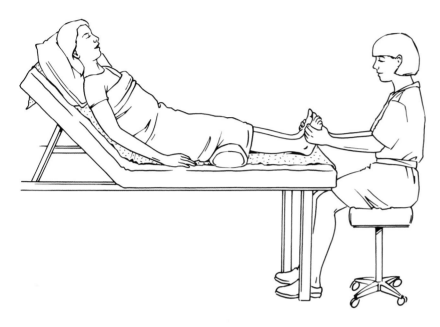

Fig. 7.1 *Light holding and centring before beginning*

REMEMBER
The location of organs and systems of the body overlap within us. Similarly when working on a particular area you will be reflexing more than one body part. When areas are tender, deciding which body part the reflex corresponds to involves discrimination and interpretation based on what the client has told you about their history and condition, and a knowledge of anatomy and physiology.

2   Observe and record the conditions of the feet.

REMEMBER
Record your observations as you work.

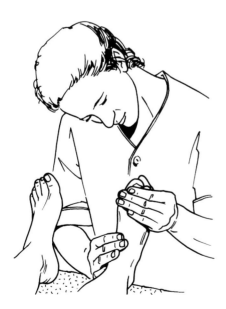

Fig. 7.2 *Observing the condition of the feet*

3   Give several relaxation techniques to both feet. Wrap up the right foot to maintain warmth, if needed.

Work the reflexes of the left foot first, then those of the right

4   Work the chest area, plantar, from diaphragm to neck line. This area includes: lungs, bronchioles, oesophagus, heart (left foot), thyroid and parathyroid glands.
5   Work the chest area, dorsal, from neck line to first metatarsal joint. Use the index or third finger and protection holds. This area includes: the upper lymphatic gland (clavicle) reflexes, the breast, and the musculature of the upper back (trapezius, rhomboids) and upper chest.

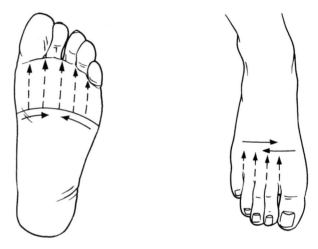

Fig. 7.3 *(a) Chest area, plantar aspect (b) Chest area, dorsal aspect*

6   Work the head-neck area, plantar, by working each toe individually. Work down from the top of the toe to the base and up from base to top. Work the front of the big toe below the nail for the nose, mouth- jaw reflexes. Work the occiput reflex on the plantar aspect of the big toe along the base of the toe pad. The head-neck area includes: sinuses, the neck, eyes, ears, pituitary, pineal, thyroid and parathyroid glands.

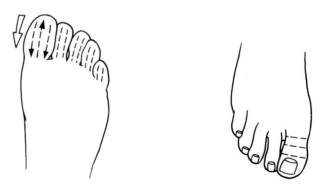

Fig. 7.4 *Head and neck areas (a) Work up and down the toes (b) Nose, mouth and jaw reflexes*

7   Work the eye and ear reflexes along the ridge at the base of the small toes.

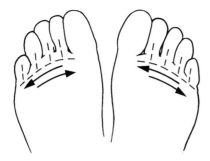

Fig. 7.5 *Eye and ear areas*

8   Work the upper abdominal cavity area reflexes, waistline to diaphragm line. This area includes: stomach, pancreas, spleen (left foot), liver (right foot), also part of the kidney, adrenal gland and transverse colon reflexes.

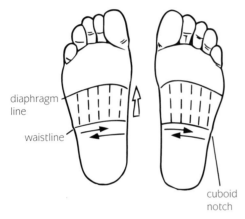

Fig. 7.6 *Upper abdominal area*

9   Work the lower abdominal cavity reflexes, heel line to waistline. This area includes: small intestine, ileo-caecal valve/appendix, ascending colon (right foot), part of the kidney and ureter, descending colon (left foot).

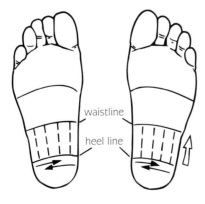

Fig. 7.7 *Lower abdominal area*

10 Work the urinary system reflexes: bladder, ureter, kidney, adrenal gland.

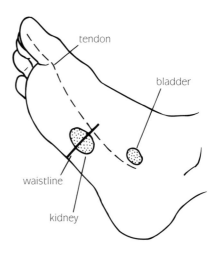

Fig. 7.8 *Urinary area, bladder to kidney*

11 Work the reproductive system reflexes near the ankles: ovary-testes (lateral), uterus-prostate (medial), fallopian tube-vas deferens/lower lymph nodes and pubis symphisus.

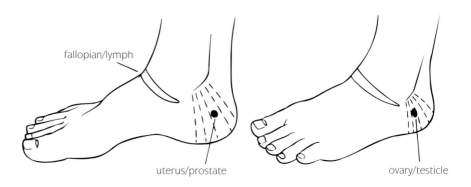

Fig. 7.9 *(a) Lymph and reproductive reflexes, medial view (b) Pelvic area and reproductive reflexes, lateral view*

12 Work the pelvic area reflexes (ankle area). This area includes: hip joint, muscles of the buttocks, lower spinal vertebrae.
13 Work the spine and major joint reflex areas. This includes the entire spine – cervical to coccyx, shoulder, arm and elbow, knee and hip.
14 Return to specific areas to give further treatment as needed.
15 Finish with solar plexus breathing-with-pressure and passive holding to end the treatment. Perform this simultaneously on both feet.

REMEMBER
Wash your hands before and after each treatment.

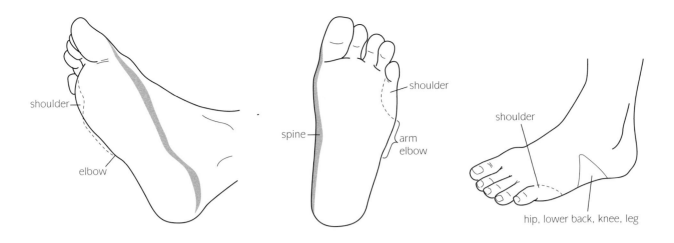

Fig. 7.10 *(a) Spine area, dorsal view (b) Spine area, plantar view, (c) Knee-leg-hip area*

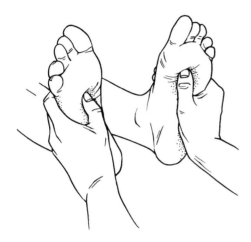

Fig. 7.11 *Solar plexus point for breathing-with-pressure*

ACTIVITY

With a partner practise this sequence (or the one given by your teacher) until you are fully competent and confident, and can relax into the treatment, while maintaining awareness.

GOOD PRACTICE

After the client rises, offer your feedback about the treatment; what the tender or congested areas relate to and what this means in terms of her health and condition. Make any suggestions about lifestyle or dietary changes as you feel appropriate. Some reflexologists like at this time to mention the possibility of certain responses to the treatment a client might feel, such as would indicate a healing process or general cleansing has been started by the body. These include possible increase in urination, a mild headache, or a little tiredness. With this knowledge, it is felt that the client will respond more positively because she understands what is going on and can work with it. However, there is a very fine line between such explanations being taken as warning, and creating anxiety, or as a suggestion which invokes the actual response, so some reflexologists do not take this approach.

Progress Check

1 Which organ reflexes are found in the chest area, dorsal and plantar?
2 Which organ reflexes are found in the neck area?
3 Which organ reflexes are found in the upper abdominal area?
4 Besides the more superficial respiratory tissues (e.g. pleura) what muscular reflexes are found on the dorsal aspect of the foot?
5 Describe clearly the location of the lower (groin) lymph nodes.

Practical aspects of treatment

> **REMEMBER**
> Reflexology is a highly adaptable therapy, simple but powerful.

How often to treat

When a client comes for help with a specific condition, treating twice a week is perhaps the ideal. However, this is not always possible so treating once a week at least is recommended as a general rule. Treatment given over several weeks, say from four to six, allows a good chance of success – though very much depends on the client's responsiveness and co-operation, and how deep-seated the condition is, because the effects of treatment are cumulative. Encouraging clients to commit to a series of regular treatments is a policy followed by many reflexologists, while others feel that this is not necessary because once a client experiences even a slight improvement she will wish to continue.

In chronic conditions, giving treatment 'little and often' brings the best results, so giving a somewhat shorter overall treatment but working on specific reflexes two or three times extra to the weekly full treatment is best where possible.

Teaching the client to work on her own reflexes between treatments means the momentum can be kept up and has the advantage of engaging the client consciously in her own healing process.

How long to treat

After the initial consultation time, treatment length varies from between 45 minutes to an hour, depending on the individual practitioner and the needs of the client. Working longer does not necessarily bring better results. The aim is to give a thorough treatment to the main reflex areas of the body and the whole of both feet, not to work every single possible reflex each time. Many reflexes are worked only when working on specific conditions related to that body part.

In circumstances other than the private clinic, it is possible to adapt treatment. For example, when working in a nursing home, or hospital or treating a friend or colleague briefly for a minor ailment, you may only work a few main or specific reflexes in the time allowed. However, be sure always to give extensive touch to the whole of both feet through your relaxation techniques.

Always work within the limits of your training and expertise.

How long to treat specific points

This will depend on such factors as the client's tolerance, the nature of the condition and the limitations of the appointment time. In general, when working specific points work on them for between 30–60 seconds, or until you and the client notice that a shift has occurred – i.e. the tenderness or congestion seems to have lessened – then give some relaxation and leave those points to continue the treatment. An alternative approach is not to work above the 60 seconds in any case and to allow the body time to absorb and respond as it will. You can then come back to these points at the end of the treatment, and touch them lightly to see how they are responding.

Adapting the treatment

Be prepared to adapt treatment to meet the special needs of your client based on such factors as age, condition, sensitivity level, congestion level, or physical or economic circumstances. Some people may be quite congested and strongly built and need a more stimulating, penetrating, vigorous type of touch. Others may be very depleted and highly sensitive and respond better to a gentler touch. You will work slightly differently on someone who is recently traumatised, perhaps by a bereavement or on someone who is depressed than you will on someone who has come for years for regular treatments and is in good health. Working in a large room in a nursing home is different from working in a private home or in a clinic setting. Be aware of all such factors and adapt your treatment accordingly.

Progress Check

1 What is a good general guide to how long to work specific reflexes?
2 What is the guiding motto when working reflexes for chronic conditions?
3 If a full treatment cannot be given, what is the best approach?

What to expect from treatment
Tender areas

Many, but not all, clients report some tenderness, soreness or pain in some reflexes. Tenderness indicates an imbalance in the flow of energy and circulation which can eventually manifest as congestion, or irritation or inflammation or weakening of the tissues. The imbalance may be quite significant and relate to or help explain the condition the client complains of. It can also not be strong enough to produce a noticeable symptom, or syndrome. A great advantage of reflexology is that it can pick up preliminary signs and give treatment so conditions need not manifest.

Tenderness can also reflect past trauma to the area, such as an operation or accident, that has healed but retains some sensitivity.

Sometimes lack of tenderness in areas associated with symptoms may not show until the third or fourth treatment as the area lacks the energy to respond. As treatments continue, the positive energy returns to them and they may become acutely sensitive before gradually normalising as treatment progresses.

Tenderness needs to be interpreted in the light of the client and individual case history.

Crystals

These are congested areas of tissue which the reflexologist can feel as tiny grains of sand under the skin or more generalised areas of lumpiness or congestion. The client may or may not experience these as tender. They also represent areas of imbalance or trauma.

Tension and variations of temperature

Some areas just feel tense or noticeably hot or cold to the reflexologist. These too represent imbalance in the reflex area.

The healing process

Sometimes a client experiences an acute episode after treatment. For example, symptoms may worsen for a short while before they improve, or she may feel extra tired, or achy for a day, or may develop a cold or sore throat. Such episodes may or may not be directly related to the treatment. Many factors in a person's life can trigger them.

However, such symptoms may result from the stimulating effects of treatment and if so, they are to be welcomed, despite temporary discomfort. They mean that the body is in the process of cleansing and healing itself. The body sometimes creates acute short-term illnesses to release toxins. This means that its immune system is strengthened and activated and can expel the negative factors within itself. Such symptoms are short-lived and will leave the client with a greater sense of well-being. All this needs explaining to the client and reassurances given, along with advice to rest and drink lots of water or herb teas to assist the process.

Keep an open mind when it comes to judging results, although the client will naturally want results as quickly as possible. Be aware that for all the good your skills are doing, if the client is not ready to change, results will not really come until she is. Also if the condition has existed for a long time, it may take a longer time to see a response, and it may be an idea to tell the client this. For yourself, as a general guide, you may expect a month of treatment for every year the condition has existed, though you need not communicate this to the client. It depends upon the individual.

Apart from your own skills, response depends on the receptivity of the client at an emotional-mental level as well as at a physical level. It all depends on the inherent vitality and strength of the system in general and whether the person is ready for change and growth. A very depleted person may take longer to recover than a basically strong person.

Do not be discouraged if you don't get amazing results with every client right away. Have patience and confidence – sometimes it seems that nothing is happening and then 'suddenly' things shift and begin to change. Much has been happening beneath the surface, but was not manifesting. The reservoir of healing energy had to be replenished before the body was ready to rid itself of the condition.

Expect the client to be discouraged at times. Expect them to experience some discomfort as well; this will depend on how toxic the body is, how much 'rubbish' has to be eliminated. They may wish to blame this on you rather than take responsibility for their own situation. While being supportive, and involved, maintain a sense of detachment from their healing process; don't lose confidence in yourself. Try to keep their outlook positive, explaining what is involved in the process and encouraging them to move forward with it.

Reflexology and medication

Bear in mind that if clients are on any drug or over-the-counter medication, especially sedatives, alcohol or nicotine, sensitivity to your touch may be reduced and effects of treatment take longer to occur. The liver processes foreign substances including medications. If the client has been on medication, the liver may need support or show signs of stress.

GOOD PRACTICE

If the client is on insulin, reflexology relaxes the body and reduces stress and this may have an effect on blood sugar levels. Make diabetic clients aware of this and ask them to inform their doctor that they are receiving treatment and to obtain written consent if possible. They are also advised to monitor their blood sugar extra carefully and report it so that in conjunction with the doctor's advice, they may be able to adjust their medication.

With other medication, especially sedatives or psychotrophic drugs, be aware that the medication may affect the client's responses. Again, eventually, as the body balances and heals itself, such medication may be reduced, but only on the advice of the doctor.

Progress Check

1   What different things can tenderness in a reflex indicate?
2   Why might a reflex which, from the case history you would expect to be tender, not register any indication of imbalance in the first one or two treatments?
3   What other indicators, besides the client's experience of tenderness, can show that an area is imbalanced?
4   What are crystals?
5   What are some signs of a healing process?
6   What do we need to bear in mind when treating clients on medication, either prescribed or over-the-counter? What cautions would you observe when treating someone on insulin therapy?

WORKING THE BODY'S REFLEXES

After working through this chapter you will be able to:

♦ locate and work the reflexes for each of the body's major systems

♦ locate and work the main back-up reflexes for each system

♦ understand how the systems inter-relate with the mind and emotions.

Once the basic techniques of reflexology have been mastered, they can be integrated into a wider application in treatment. As well as giving the basic whole body treatment to discover the body's weak or imbalanced areas, a reflexologist also gives specific treatment to the areas most involved in the imbalances, either directly or indirectly: the organ systems of the body's physiology. It is useful for students to have an understanding of the reflexes, system by system and this chapter serves as a reference for the reflexes to consider working for certain conditions. It can be cross-referenced with Appendix 1 on Common Conditions. When treating the reflexes for these systems, try to keep in mind that we are treating them in order to help the body do what it is naturally trying to do – perform its functions in an optimal way.

This chapter is not intended as a substitute for the detailed study of anatomy and physiology required of a professional reflexologist; such study is a separate aspect of training beyond the scope of this book. The introductions to each system given here are intended to put that system into a holistic context.

Reflexes for the nervous system

Communication, response, movement

The nervous system is the body's primary communication network, mediating between sensations and the body's reactions to them, and also motivating all of the body's movements, both voluntary and involuntary. In addition the nerves work in conjunction with the endocrine glands to maintain the body's immunity, homeostasis, and its response to – and recovery from – stress.

This system represents the organism's sensitivity to its internal and external surroundings and its mechanisms for relating to them and adjusting to them. It is in essence the energy of air which ideally moves freely and smoothly, and is grounded in regularity or rhythm. When air energy is ungrounded, there is lack of concentration, a spacey feeling, loss of memory or consciousness. When this flow of air energy is blocked or congested it results in such things as tension, numbness, tingling, spasm, paralysis, pain, arrhythmia.

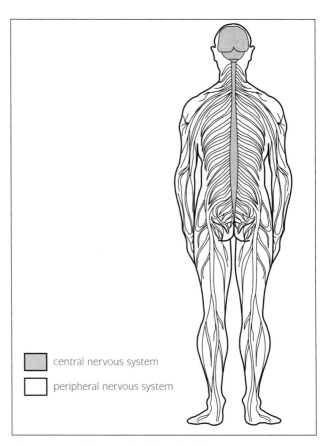

Fig. 8.1 *(a) The central and peripheral nervous systems*

central nervous system

peripheral nervous system

Pain is the body's communication that there is something wrong; such pain may also be referred, i.e. pain caused in one area can appear in another part of the body. Pain is a hyper-state of nerve activity, but prolonged or chronic pain can also weaken and deplete the body's energy.

Deep abdominal breathing nourishes our energy. Deep relaxation allows it to flow freely.

Reflexes for the nervous system
These include:

- diaphragm – solar plexus
- spine: cervical, thoracic, lumbar, sacrum, coccyx for nerves of the autonomic nervous system to organs (the sympathetic and parasympathetic)
- brain for co-ordination between the central and autonomic systems
- brain for cranial nerves to sense organs
- sense organs for eyes, ears, nose, tongue (mouth)
- individual muscle groups and areas for peripheral nerves in those areas, e.g. face for trigeminal nerve, shoulder for brachial plexus, lumbar-5, sacrum, pelvis, sciatic reflexes for sciatic nerve problems.

THE AUTONOMIC NERVOUS SYSTEM

parts affected	para-sympathetic	sympathetic	general result
pupils	contracted	dilated	controls the amount of light entering the eyes
cilary muscles	contracted	relaxed	controls accommodation of the eye
blood vessels	arterioles of glands and viscera dilated	arterioles of alimentary canal and skin con-stricted; those of skeletal muscles dilated or constricted by different fibres; tone raised in walls of larger vessels	adjusts the blood pressure and the distribution of the blood
spleen	dilated	constricted	adjusts the quality and quantity of blood in circulation
heart beat	slowed and weakened	hastened and strengthened	adjusts the rate of the heart according to the blood pressure and varying muscle activity
bronchioles	constricted	dilated	adjusts ease of breathing to requirements
sweat glands		activity increased	produces extra sweat in anticipation of heat production during activity
adrenal medulla		activity increased	reinforces direct effects mentioned above
peristalsis of the alimen-tary canal	increased	decreased	controls the speed of passage of food and the rate of digestion
sphincters	relaxed	contracted	
digestive glands	activity increased	activity decreased	*note*: digestion is slow when body activity is great and vice versa

Fig. 8.1 *(b) The autonomic nervous system*

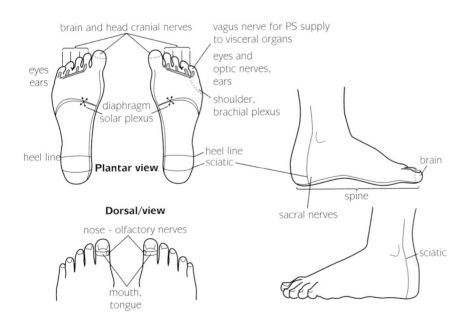

Fig. 8.1 *(c) Reflexes for the nervous system*

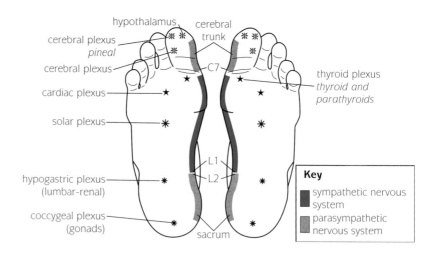

Fig. 8.1 *(d) The reflexes of the autonomic nervous system*
Adapted with kind permission of Association Reflex Therapy Total Faure-Alderson

Reflexes for the immune system

Preservation of individual vital force

Believing prevention is better than cure, reflexology recognises that when the vital force is strong the body can usually overcome disease organisms. The strength and integrity of the immune system is a reflection of the vital force.

Immunity epitomises the concept of 'holistic' because it involves the whole body and the body's relationship with its environment. The immunity exists in each cell – our cellular immunity – and also in bodily fluids and processes – our humoural immunity. It involves hormones, lymphatic cells, the blood transportation system, nerves, organs like the liver and spleen, and chemicals such as neurotransmitters. When the body is congested, when it is weakened by repeated stress, when waste is allowed to build up in the body – either physically through poor nutrition and poor elimination, or emotionally or mentally in the form of unwanted or unneeded feelings and attitudes – immunity becomes compromised because a 'ground' is created in which pathogens can thrive, tissues degenerate. Vital strength can be nourished and protected by a more positive lifestyle.

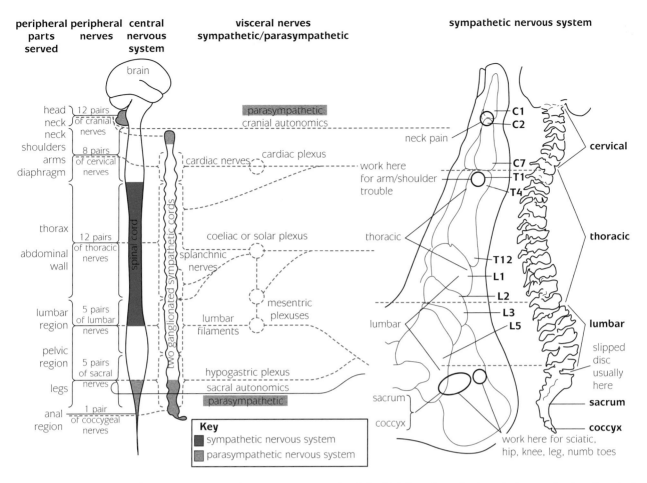

Fig. 8.2 *(a) The sympathetic and parasympathetic nervous systems*

Fig. 8.2 *(b) The reflexes for the spinal nerves leaving the spinal cord (Additional material courtesy of Association Reflex Therapy Total Faure-Alderson)*

Reflexes for the immune system include:

♦ endocrine glands: pineal, pituitary, thymus, thyroid, parathyroid, adrenal, pancreatic, ovaries and testicles
♦ nervous system
♦ eliminative channels, lymphatics, and the liver
♦ spleen.

> **ACTIVITY**
> Practise working the reflexes for the immune system. As you work visualise the anatomy and function of each part as it affects the whole.

Reflexes for the endocrine system

Communication, balance and integrity

The endocrine glands secrete hormones into the bloodstream. 'Hormone' derives from a Greek word meaning to stir up or urge on and each hormone carries a message to a particular organ or cell,

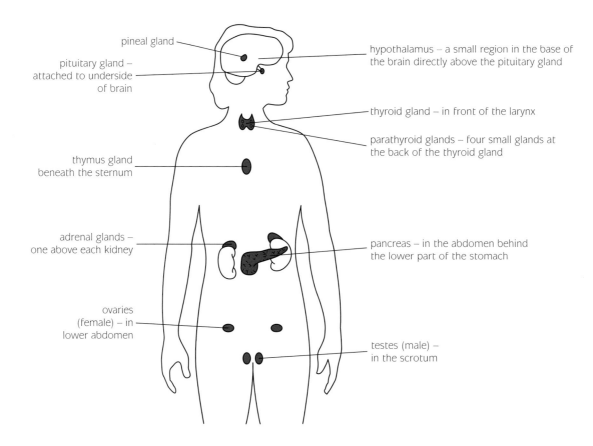

Fig. 8.3 *(a) The endocrine system*

stimulating its function in a certain way and keeping it in tune with what the rest of the body is doing. The endocrine glands help maintain homeostasis, a sense of integrity and a balance of functions. They integrate the organism's various functions into one finely tuned whole.

Functions of hormones

- In close co-operation with the nervous system, hormones enhance our inner communication and balance, so vital for both dynamic activity and restful calm.
- As part of the immune system, they enable us to both respond to and recover from stress and pathogenic challenges.
- As part of the reproductive system, hormone secretions provide smooth and healthy functioning of these vital organs.

ACTIVITY

Research the activity of each endocrine gland and what each of the hormones does in the body.

Gland	Hormone
Pineal gland	melatonin, adrenoglomerulotropin
Pituitary gland	GH, MSH, TSH, ACTH, ADH, FSH, LH, prolactin, oxytocin
Thyroid gland	thyroxin, tri-iodo-thyronine, calcitonin, oxytocin, anti-diuretic
Parathyroid glands	parathyroid hormones
Thymus gland	thymosin, thymic humoural factor, thymic factor, thymopoetin
The islets of Langerhorn (pancreas)	glucagon, insulin
Adrenal glands	mineral corticoids, gluco-corticoids, gonado-corticoids, adrenaline, noradrenalin
Ovaries	oestrogen, progesterone, relaxin
Testes	testosterone, inhibin

The reflexes for the endocrine system

- pineal gland
- pituitary gland
- thyroid gland and helper to thyroid
- thymus gland
- islets of Langerhorn/pancreas
- adrenal glands
- reproductive glands: ovaries and testes

Back-up reflexes for the endocrine system

- nerves to these glands
- blood and lymph circulation reflexes
- diaphragm

REMEMBER

For any type of stress or shock always include the endocrine gland reflexes as well as the immune system, nervous system reflexes, and relaxation reflexes.

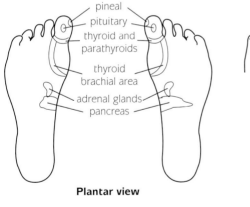

Plantar view

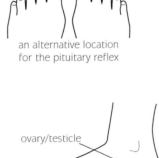

an alternative location for the pituitary reflex

Lateral view

REMEMBER

The endocrine system links with the nervous and lymphatic systems to form the immune system, and with the reproductive system

Fig. 8.3 *(b) Reflexes for the endocrine system*

ACTIVITY

Practise working each of the reflexes for the endocrine system.
Visualise their anatomy and functions as you work.

Reflexes for the respiratory system

Rhythm of life, stream of consciousness

Without the breath of life we would not live for more than a few minutes, hence breathing is the primary vital function. The respiratory system receives the nourishing vital force as air. It has a dual life-saving function: providing oxygen for cells' metabolic functions and eliminating their carbon dioxide waste. The lungs nourish and they cleanse. Through the nasal passages the respiratory system forms a first line of defence against airborne pathogens.

Breathing is a rhythmic activity, closely related to the heart's rhythmic contractions. Blood passes from heart to lungs for oxygenation before returning to circulation. The depth and rhythm of the breathing is intimately connected to the nervous system, to our emotions, and our mental awareness. Breathing is in a sense the physical manifestation of our consciousness. Emotional and mental issues, for example fear and anxiety, can both influence and reflect breathing. Conversely – as the yogis of India have long known – we can influence our emotions and our mental states, our response to stress, indeed our entire health by learning deep, rhythmic, calm breathing.

> **REMEMBER**
> The respiratory system links with the nervous system, the quality of blood and lymph, heart rhythm and the endocrine system.

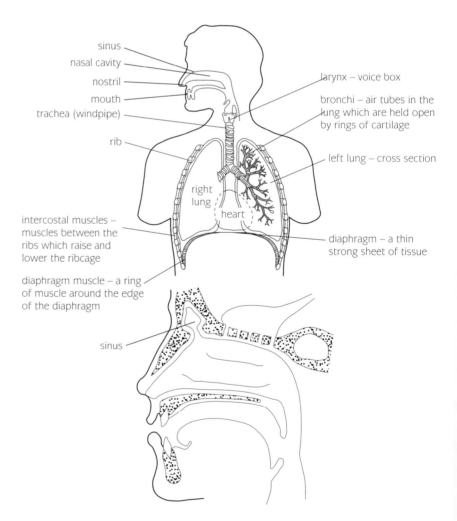

Fig. 8.4 *(a) The respiratory system*

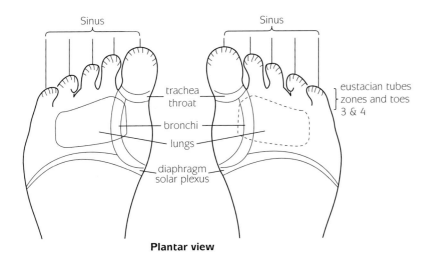

Plantar view

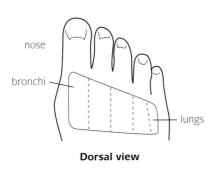

Dorsal view

Fig. 8.4 *(b) Reflexes for the respiratory system*

Reflexes for the respiratory system

- ◆ nose
- ◆ eustachian tubes
- ◆ trachea
- ◆ lungs: bronchial tubes zone 1, alveoli zones 2, 3
- ◆ diaphragm and solar plexus

Back-up reflexes

- ◆ lymphatic reflexes
- ◆ ileo-caecal valve
- ◆ stomach
- ◆ nerves T 1–3

REMEMBER
A tense diaphragm muscle can inhibit full breathing.

ACTIVITY
Practise working the reflexes for the respiratory system. Visualise the anatomy as you work. Research and understand the influence each back-up reflex can have on the respiratory system.

Reflexes for the lymphatic system

Ocean of life: nourishing, cleansing, protecting

The lymphatic system is intimately connected with all systems and functions: with the cardio-vascular function, with cell metabolism, with immunity, with nutrition, with glandular secretions, with bone and nerve. It is an aspect of the water element and is like an ocean of life-giving fluid in which all our cells are floating and through which they receive nourishment and are relieved of their wastes.

Lymph fluid is a viscous, straw-coloured liquid like honey. This fluid is transported through special vessels of different sizes and pauses at lymph

> **REMEMBER**
> The lymphatic system links with the nervous, endocrine and circulatory systems and with every cell of the body.

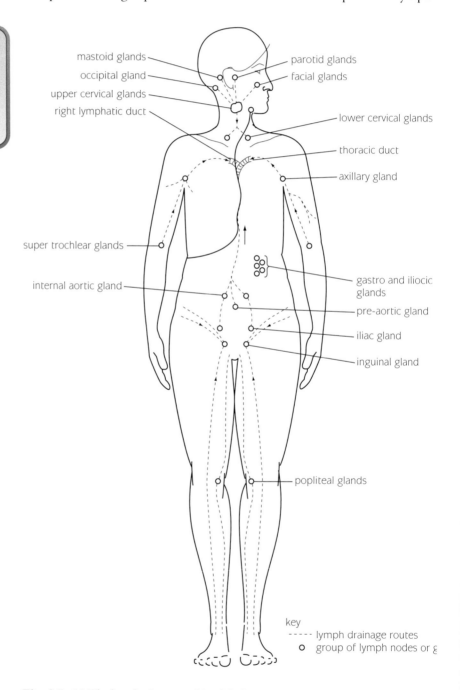

Fig. 8.5 *(a) The lymphatic system (simplified)*

nodes for filtering, and fighting infection by lymph immune cells. Lymph lacteals in the small intestine aid in the absorption of nutrients. Lymph fluid around cells interconnects with blood capillaries, carrying in nutrients, removing cell waste.

Reflexes for the lymphatic system
- neck for cervical nodes
- throat for tonsils and adenoids
- base of toes, dorsal, for clavicle lymph nodes
- breasts for mamillary glands
- chest zone 1 for thymus gland
- shoulder for axilla lymph nodes
- anterior malleoli for groin lymph nodes
- spleen
- small intestine for lymph lacteals

> **REMEMBER**
> Always work the lymphatic reflexes as part of the immune system and when helping to strengthen the immune system. The lymph is one of the five eliminative channels and a little attention to it at each treatment helps keep the body's balance of functions healthy.

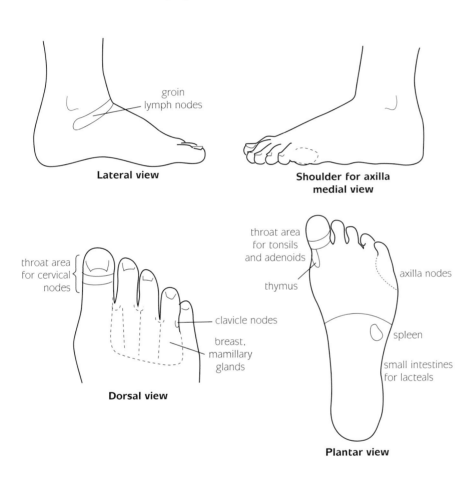

Fig. 8.5 (b) Reflexes for the lymphatic system

Back-up for the lymphatic system
- adrenals
- liver
- heart and blood circulation
- immune reflexes

Reflexes for the urinary system

Waters of life
The urinary system is one of the eliminative channels of the body. The kidneys help purify the blood and maintain its correct balance of acid and alkaline. They symbolise the balance of the water element in the body as emotional balance, selecting what is good to conserve and rejecting what is not needed as we relate to others. Water is inherently cool and heavy, and is needed to cool the acid heat of blood and as the base fluid to promote reproduction and growth. It is a stabilising, life-promoting influence. However, if it becomes dammed up to excess or depleted to deficiency, it can provoke tension, irritability, worry, fear and anxiety. If isolated from the warmth of loving and caring, water can become cold and unable to nurture. Good kidney function supports good cardio-vascular function through purifying the blood and influencing blood pressure. The kidneys influence the lower extremities, lower back and legs, the motivation to move through life with either ease or dis-ease and discomfort.

The bladder is also connected to the stress response and can react to emotions to do with stress such as fear and anxiety.

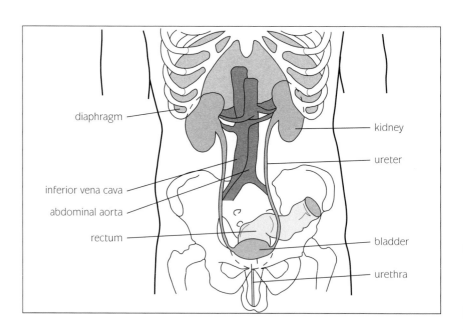

Fig. 8.6 *(a) The urinary system*

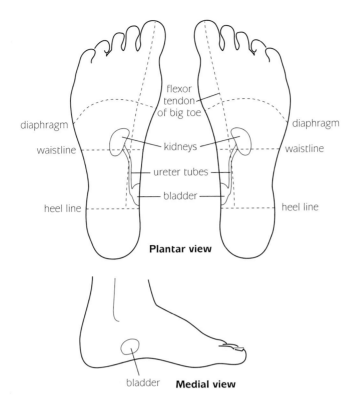

Fig. 8.6 *(b) Reflexes for the urinary system*

Reflexes for the urinary system
- kidneys
- ureter
- bladder

Back-up reflexes
- glands
- the nerves supplying the kidneys and bladder
- diaphragm and stress reflexes

REMEMBER
The urinary system is one of the five eliminative channels of the body and a little attention to it at each treatment helps keep the body's balance of functions healthy.

ACTIVITY
Research which glands influence kidney activity and the role the kidneys play in regulating blood pressure. Practise working the reflexes for the urinary system. Visualise the system's anatomy as you work.

GOOD PRACTICE

When working the ureter to kidney reflex and the kidney reflex, remember to relax the tendon as you work over it. Kidney reflexes are often tender on some people, so proceed cautiously over this reflex.

Reflexes for the digestive system

We are what we eat

The digestive system is our central channel from which nutrition flows out to every cell, tissue and organ. While good food is important, equally important is whether that food is fully digested and assimilated to release its energy. If this function fails, we do not derive the energy we need from food; useless residues accumulate, which may become toxic, the body has to use extra energy to expel or contain them. Disturbed digestion can create potentially toxic matter which becomes the ground cause of disease in various body parts. Many people experience relief

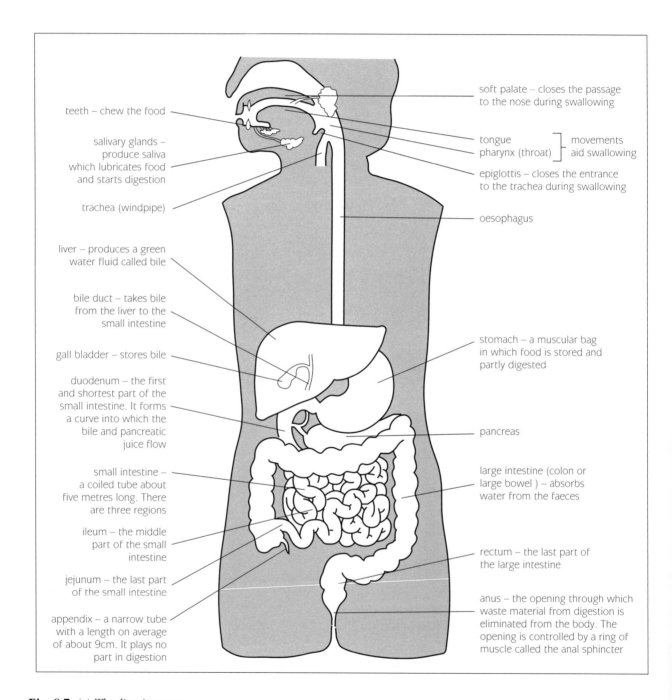

teeth – chew the food

salivary glands – produce saliva which lubricates food and starts digestion

trachea (windpipe)

liver – produces a green water fluid called bile

bile duct – takes bile from the liver to the small intestine

gall bladder – stores bile

duodenum – the first and shortest part of the small intestine. It forms a curve into which the bile and pancreatic juice flow

small intestine – a coiled tube about five metres long. There are three regions

ileum – the middle part of the small intestine

jejunum – the last part of the small intestine

appendix – a narrow tube with a length on average of about 9cm. It plays no part in digestion

soft palate – closes the passage to the nose during swallowing

tongue
pharynx (throat) — movements aid swallowing

epiglottis – closes the entrance to the trachea during swallowing

oesophagus

stomach – a muscular bag in which food is stored and partly digested

pancreas

large intestine (colon or large bowel) – absorbs water from the faeces

rectum – the last part of the large intestine

anus – the opening through which waste material from digestion is eliminated from the body. The opening is controlled by a ring of muscle called the anal sphincter

Fig. 8.7 *(a) The digestive system*

from their symptoms simply by adopting a cleansing diet or fast which simultaneously improves digestion and allows the body to eliminate waste which otherwise can seep into tissues from the digestive tract. Digestion in the stomach and small intestines represents the fire element, while in the colon it embodies the earth element, nourishing solidity and groundedness.

Organs such as the liver, pancreas and gall bladder play important parts in the digestive process and their healthy functioning is also necessary to good digestion.

Digestion is greatly influenced by the environment in which we eat. Eating with a calm mind and emotions and a positive outlook enhances digestion and assimilation. The colon is also influenced by our state of mind and emotions, as well as by such things as sleep and exercise. Good food, good digestion, good elimination along with mental-emotional calm are important for a healthy digestive system.

Reflexes for the digestive system

- mouth for digestive enzymes
- oesophagus
- stomach
- small intestine
- liver and gall bladder
- pancreas
- large intestine, ileo-caecal valve
- sigmoid and rectum

REMEMBER
The digestive system links to respiration, lymph and blood, the autonomic nervous function, endocrine system, and mental-emotional states.

REMEMBER
The colon eliminates a large proportion of bodily waste. Working it at each treatment helps keep the body's balance of functions healthy.

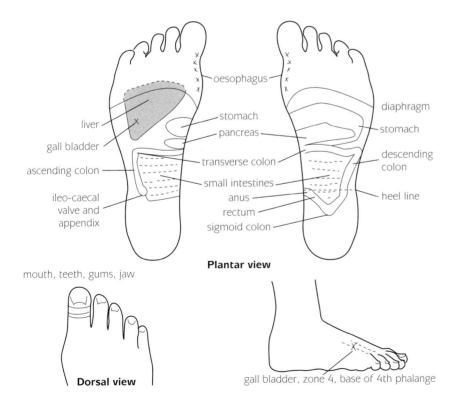

Fig. 8.7 (b) Reflexes for the digestive system

Back-up reflexes

- diaphragm
- chronic area at Achilles heel
- nerves to the digestive organs
- stress reflexes

Reflexes for the reproductive system

Source of life

The reproductive system includes the glands secreting hormones which affect it. Health of the reproductive organs is important for bringing forth new life. It also influences the health of the body as a whole. In a sense our own life is a series of births and deaths, of rites of passage as we grow from one stage to another. At each stage we leave behind some things, as we are reborn to new ideas, new possibilities.

Life which does not continue to grow and develop, withers and dies. The energy for continuing transformation and growth comes in a sense from our reproductive organs, which hold the essence and reserves of the vital force. Our sense of identity is linked to our gender and sexuality; a healthy sense of self-esteem is reflected in positive loving relationships, and physically as strong immunity. Even minor problems in the cycles of reproductive organs can influence our overall health, draining our energy. The healthy functioning of the sex organs plays a part in retarding the ageing process and allows us to grow into our older years in a positive state of health and mind.

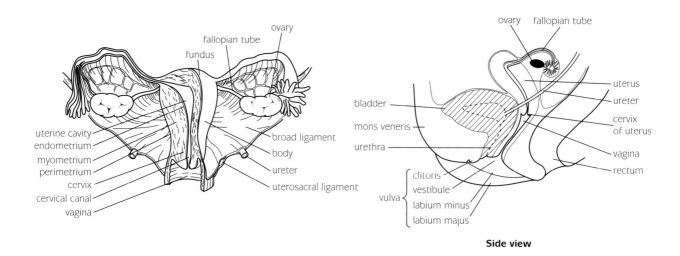

Fig. 8.8 *(a) The female reproductive system*

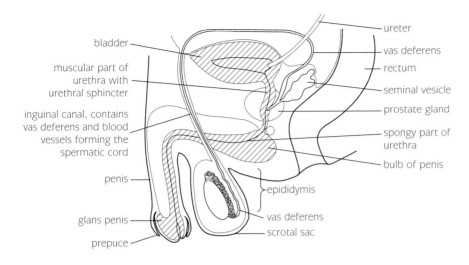

Fig. 8.8 *(b) The male reproductive system*

Reflexes for the reproductive organs

- pituitary gland
- adrenal glands
- breast
- ovaries and testes
- fallopian tubes and vas deferens
- uterus
- prostate

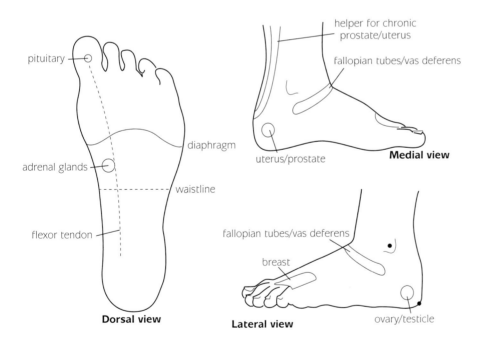

Fig. 8.8 *(c) Reflexes for the reproductive system*

Back-up reflexes

- nerves for these glands and organs
- kidney-bladder
- lymphatic reflexes

- colon
- liver
- chronic/Achilles tendon area

ACTIVITY

Research the mechanism through which stress can affect the reproductive function. Practise working the reflexes for the reproductive system. Visualise the system's anatomy as you work.

Reflexes for the musculo-skeletal system

Structure of life

This system, which can seem somewhat hard and disconnected from the other vital functions of the organism, is nevertheless just as intimately involved with the workings of the whole as any other. Structure governs function.

Marrow within bones is necessary for the health of the lymph and thus the entire immune system. Bones combine the solidity of earth with the lightness of air as internally they are a matrix of spaces. Similarly muscle tissue is solid but enlivened by nerves, nourished and cleansed with blood and lymph. Muscles need both exercise and rest, stretching and relaxing, nutrition and waste removal. The heart is a muscle organ and has the needs of any other muscle to keep it healthy.

The spine provides a structure and by its flexibility and balance allows freedom of communication and movement among all other systems. Stiffness and rigidity, tension and pain in the joints affects the whole. We can think of our spine as like a golden thread which dangles to the ground, but whose origin comes from above. We are in a sense hanging on that golden thread as we pass through life and we need only touch the ground lightly leaving muscles relaxed, nerves free to move us gracefully and easily through life.

Reflexes for the musculo-skeletal system
- spine: cervical, thoracic, lumbar, sacrum-coccyx, nerves and muscles attaching to the spine
- shoulder
- arm, elbow
- neck
- hip
- hip-knee-leg
- pelvic muscles
- sciatic area
- chronic sciatica area (Achilles area)
- diaphragm
- heart
- dorsal chest area – muscles of the upper back

REMEMBER

The muscular-skeletal system links with the quality of blood and lymph, to the nervous and endocrine systems, to the heart and eliminative organs.

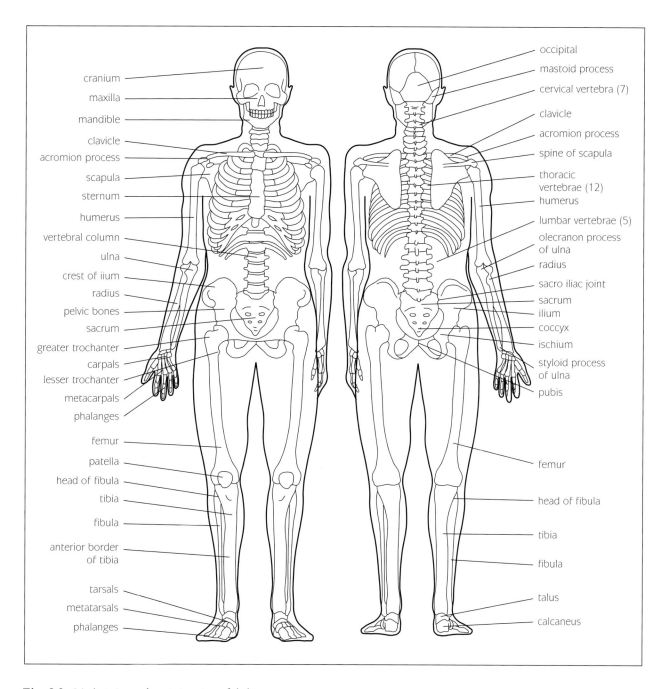

Fig. 8.9 *(a) Anterior and posterior view of skeleton*

Back-up reflexes
- adrenals
- kidneys
- parathyroids
- elimination channels

ACTIVITY

Practise working the reflexes for the musculo-skeletal system.
Visualise the system's anatomy in the body as you work.

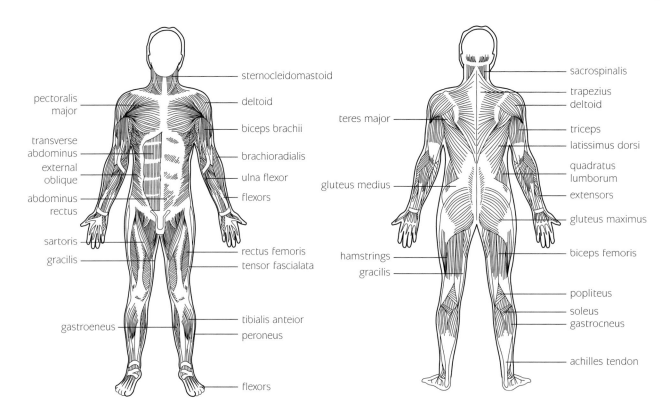

Fig. 8.9 (b) The muscular system (superficial muscles)

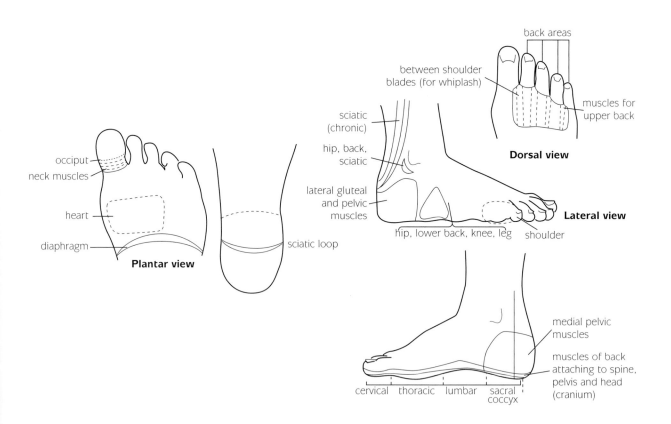

Fig. 8.9 (c) Reflexes for the musculo-skeletal system

Reflexes for the cardio-vascular system

River of life

The cardio-vascular system is greatly influenced by the work of other organs such as the kidneys and the liver, as well as the nerves and glands. Our blood is literally our river of life, the transport system which carries oxygen, nutrients, enzymes, neurotransmitters and immune factors to cells, and removes metabolic wastes. Its warmth and life reflect the fire element. When blood carries impurities, it will naturally weaken the healthy functioning of cells and tissues. When obstructions such as plaque on vessel walls, or weak vessels impair the flow, the heart muscle must work ever harder to supply blood to the body. The heart and blood symbolise the joy of life, the optimism of spring, and the courage to face the challenges of life. The heart, in its rhythmic emptying and filling and giving forth symbolises our loving relationships with others, whether we are open to receiving and giving love.

Reflexes for the cardio-vascular system

- heart
- lungs
- diaphragm
- liver

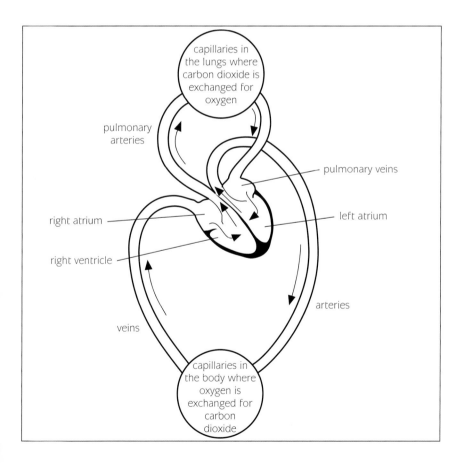

Fig. 8.10 *(a) The cardio-vascular system*

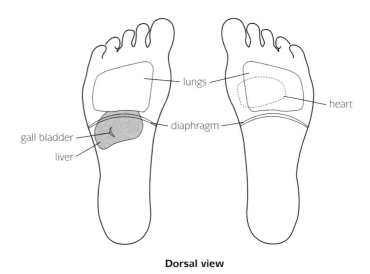

Dorsal view

Fig. 8.10 *(b) Reflexes for the cardio-vascular system*

Back-up reflexes
- kidneys – adrenals
- large intestine
- nerves to heart and organs
- thyroid gland
- leg and cross reflexes for varicose veins, phlebitis

ACTIVITY

Research and understand the influence the liver, kidneys and diaphragm have on the healthy functioning of the heart and blood. Research and understand how the stress response can increase blood pressure and how repeated stress can lead to primary hypertension. Practise working the reflexes for the cardio-vascular system. Visualise the anatomy of the system as you work.

Reflexes for the skin

The living surface

The skin, or integument system, is the largest vital organ of the body. It performs a multitude of complex functions necessary to life and health. The skin is evolved from the same embryonic cells as are the kidneys and the lungs – disturbances in the functioning of these three organs often influence each other. When the eliminative functions of the kidneys and lungs are under par, the skin is used as the organ through which the body tries to eliminate the excess waste. Liver function also influences the skin. The health of the skin thus reflects the health of the inner body.

Because the skin covers the entire body, there are no specific reflexes for it, but we work the organs and systems which influence it.

Reflexes for the skin

- kidneys
- liver
- lung
- adrenals
- large intestine
- lymphatic reflexes
- endocrine reflexes
- nervous system and diaphragm-solar plexus
- blood and circulatory system

ACTIVITY

Practise working the reflexes for the skin. As you work, visualise how each of the organs and systems affects the health of the skin.

9 SOME SPECIAL APPLICATIONS OF REFLEXOLOGY

After working through this chapter you will be able to:

◆ understand the special considerations and adaptations involved in treating children, pregnant women, elderly clients, clients with disabilities, psychiatric problems, HIV-AIDS, or drug addiction

◆ understand the value of teaching clients self-reflexology

◆ recognise the special considerations necessary when giving reflexology in hospitals

◆ appreciate the importance of knowing about care provided in your local community and the value of being able to pass this information to your clients.

The basic reflexology techniques and treatments outlined in the previous chapters can be applied to a variety of clients, with different conditions and in many locations. This chapter seeks to focus on a few of these variations and give some extra guidance on how to approach and adapt treatment. These can only be basic guidelines and suggestions. Using reflexology in some of these areas is relatively new and much useful knowledge is still unfolding.

The chapter also looks at some of the community care and support available for clients. Reflexologists can often give their clients additional help by making them aware that such support is available.

Reflexology for children

> **REMEMBER**
> The most important factor in the happy, healthy development of a child is the love from adults which engenders a sense of security and self-esteem. Without security, the child experiences fear and necessarily builds defences to protect herself. Without the fundamental acceptance which builds self-esteem, she cannot be in turn loving and accepting of others.

Treating children with reflexology is both effective for the client and highly rewarding for the practitioner. Children are liable to be much more responsive to treatment than adults as their bodies are still relatively 'open', have not yet become fixed in self-protecting or negative patterns and are less toxic than ours, though there are always exceptions to this. Each child must be understood as an individual.

Children's inquisitive minds make them naturally open to the discovery that reflexology can have a gentle but effective influence on their health.

Reflexology's advantages for treating children
◆ It is a non-invasive, hence non-threatening treatment.
◆ Touching the feet may be acceptable whereas touching other parts of the body may be inappropriate. It can be helpful not only in physical but also emotional conditions. Teaching parents to give reflexology can enhance open communication and nurturing.
◆ It is gentle and can be made 'fun' to do.
◆ It gives children a positive body-image.

Reflexology may be particularly advantageous in helping children who have been abused or orphaned or are otherwise emotionally damaged. It can give them the comfort and security they need from a loving touch coming from unconditional regard for their welfare, helping to rebuild their self-esteem.

Points to consider when treating children

1   Try to make treatments enjoyable; introduce an element of play into them. This does not mean tickling the feet, but rather in different ways making the treatments fun. For example, depending on age, you might encourage them to bring in a favourite doll or soft toy to have treatment too and you can show the child how to treat his or her doll or teddy. Think up a few verbal games for older children, perhaps related to their understanding of the body's organs. They can benefit from visualisations.

2   Remember that children's bones are soft and still growing. Handle the feet gently, with extra care.

3   Children's feet are likely to be more sensitive and although a generally firm touch is needed to avoid tickling, it need not be deep. For very young infants simply a gentle stroking is enough.

4   Gear the length of treatment to the age and attention span of the child. Don't go on so long that the child becomes uninterested. It is not necessary to treat absolutely every possible point on the feet, as long as the necessary ones and their back-ups are treated and the feet are touched in general in all parts.

5   A parent's permission must be obtained. Depending on the age of the child, the parent may or may not be invited to attend the treatment session. A parent's presence can be an advantage, enabling the therapist to educate the parent about the treatment and show them how to perform simple reflexology between treatments if this is appropriate. On the other hand, some older children may not wish their parents to be present and this needs to be respected.

6   Parents must always be fully informed of your findings and recommendations. It is their responsibility to decide how much to inform the child. You must discuss this subject with the parent before treatment begins so that you will know how to approach it with the child.

7   When treating babies, be sure to treat the mother, or primary nurturer, as well. Her well-being will be transferred to the infant. Her imbalances may be a factor in the baby's condition. This could apply to older children as well but is particularly important in treating infants.

8   When treating girls and boys approaching puberty, again careful assessment must be made. Reflexes in the genito-urinary areas may be tender but this does not indicate abnormal function, merely that the organs are naturally more active at this time. They need only a mild treatment.

9   If treating children in special homes or hospitals, try to arrange as much privacy as possible during sessions.

Some ailments of childhood that can benefit from reflexology include: colic and stomach troubles, sleep disturbance, incontinence, ear and respiratory problems, allergies, hyperactivity, learning disabilities, sluggishness, skin problems, and menstrual problems in puberty.

ACTIVITY

Arrange to give a talk to a group of new mothers or pregnant women, such as the National Childbirth Trust or La Leche League. While informing them of reflexology, listen to their experiences about their children's ailments. Make a list of any points new to you which you will need to bear in mind when treating children.

Progress Check

1 What precautions do you need to remember when treating young children?
2 Why is it a good idea to treat the mother as well as the baby for problems in infancy?
3 Why might reproductive reflexes in puberty be sensitive even though the child is healthy and developing normally?
4 Why is only gentle stroking needed when treating young infants?

Reflexology for elders

Categorising people as elders or elderly is not as straightforward as it first appears. Some senior citizens are thoroughly robust, healthy and active while others are burdened with chronic diseases. Try not to assume all elderly people are victims but aim to support their sense of power over their lives, within any existing constraints. Each person must be assessed on an individual basis. Reflexology can help to inhibit ageing processes and relieve many minor problems that interfere with the sense of well-being.

Some of the factors which naturally slow down or weaken in older years are: circulation, glandular function, immunity. Some older people may be prone to excessive worry, irritation, or depression. This will have its effect on the body, especially the kidney and liver; sleep patterns may be disturbed.

Reflexology's advantages for treating elderly clients
- It is non-invasive, non-threatening, gentle but effective.
- It provides a positive experience of touch which can too often be lacking in the client's life; this has positive consequences on many levels.
- Depending on the client's state, it can be taught to them, providing them with a positive role in their own health care and in the relief of symptoms.

- Given regularly twice a year it can help tone body functions and enhance well-being, even when there are no specific complaints.

Points to consider when treating elderly clients

1 Bones may be brittle and joints both stiffer and more liable to injury; toes on the feet may be locked in position. Likewise, the skin may be very weak and thin, circulation poor and capillaries weak, and bruising may occur easily; healing from any injury takes much longer in these circumstances. Feet must be handled with due care. Touch may need to be lighter. Work within the limitations of the client's range of movement, use no force, allow flexibility to increase gradually where possible.

2 Session length needs to be related to the condition of the client. Short but frequent sessions may be called for, especially in chronic conditions. 'Little but often' is the key.

3 Adjust expectations to the situation. Long-standing chronic conditions may not show an obvious response for a considerable time. The treatment is still having a positive effect.

4 When working in nursing homes, hospitals or with clients whose mental faculties are compromised, you need to obtain the permission of the doctor in charge or the client's guardian before beginning treatment. It helps if you can interest the staff in reflexology. Explain the treatment and encourage them to reinforce any recommendations you make.

5 Any medication the client is taking may influence the effects of the treatment, the client's level of sensitivity or the client's perception of the effects. Find out what medication is being taken and what its effects are likely to be, and adjust your treatment accordingly. Inform the physician, nurse or family member that treatment may influence the body so that medication needs to be monitored.

Reflexes of particular importance in elderly clients, no matter what their condition, include: stress and immune reflexes, glands, circulation, brain reflexes, eliminative channels, adrenals for muscle tone, spine for flexibility and nerve supply.

> **REMEMBER**
> Holistic principles such as treating the client as an individual, enhancing the vital force, encouraging client engagement with treatment apply to elderly clients as much as to any other.

> **GOOD PRACTICE**
> Handle the client's feet with care and concern. Obtain permission of the client's physician or guardian if circumstances require it.

ACTIVITY

Arrange to give a talk to a nursing home staff about reflexology. While there observe the conditions that potential clients live in: be alert to such factors as schedules of eating, sleeping, bathing, how clients' time is occupied. Ask the audience for the benefit of their experience in treating elderly patients. Make a list of points to remember when working in such homes and when treating clients in them. Educate staff to the benefits of reflexology to them in terms of relief of stress, health maintenance and 'care for the carer'.

> 1 What is the advantage of treatment which is 'little-but-often'?
> 2 Why is it necessary to handle the feet of elderly clients with particular care? What are you trying to avoid?
> 3 How can reflexology help with elderly clients' tendency to excessive worry?
> 4 In what ways can reflexology benefit already fit and healthy elderly clients?

Reflexology for pregnancy and childbirth

While pregnancy is part of the natural cycle and women's bodies are equipped and adapted to experience it successfully, pregnancy is also a period when life and death are very close, both for mother and foetus. Pregnancy also places particular demands on the emotions as well as the body of the mother. So while taking a positive attitude towards it as a natural condition, therapists must also be aware that difficulties may arise which can make it uncomfortable for the mother or even threaten its natural progression to a healthy outcome for mother and child.

Reflexology given in pregnancy can not only help improve the mother's overall health but can shorten the length of labour and promote a healthier outcome for mother and baby. No doubt the baby in the womb is also feeling the healing effects of reflexology. Bear in mind, however, that pregnancy is not the time to undergo cleansing or treatment for other conditions. During pregnancy, treatment can be general, aiming to raise the overall health of the whole body without any particular emphasis on the reproductive reflexes until the last six weeks of pregnancy.

Understand the unique features of pregnancy and bear in mind the following cautions, while working within your own range of expertise.

> **REMEMBER**
> Treat the mother holistically, with due care for her individual situation and condition. Treatment given before conception can improve fertility, the overall health of the mother and father and thus that of the child.

- If there is history of miscarriage, you may not wish to give treatment in the first trimester, until the pregnancy is well established. Obtain the physician's advice and written consent.
- If this is a first pregnancy or previous pregnancy has been normal, some reflexologists feel some treatment may be given during the first trimester but only treating generally, avoiding reproductive reflexes. Many reflexologists feel it is very important to avoid treatment during this time altogether in case, should anything untoward occur, the practitioner may be blamed.

Common ailments that occur and relate to pregnancy include: nausea, constipation, fatigue, water retention, headaches, disturbed sleep, leg cramps, back ache, sore breasts, worry and depression. As pregnancy progresses extra strains are placed on the mother's posture and circulation which may cause problems either before or after the birth. Reflexology can help with these.

As a student it is not advisable to practise on pregnant clients, both for your own and the client's safety and well-being. Once you have fully completed your training and gained your qualification, you may consider extending your practice to these clients as your experience grows.

ACTIVITY

Research and understand the more serious possible complications of pregnancy. Make a list of reflexes you would consider working to help with these problems within a general treatment.

Ensure the client is in a comfortable position, with back and knees supported. Treatment may even be given with client lying on her side. Change the client's position according to need, stage of pregnancy and state of circulation.

Childbirth

Reflexology given during pregnancy can shorten the time of labour. Given during labour it can help relieve the mother's fatigue and pain – if it is a welcomed touch. Some women react differently to touch in labour than they do at other times. Fathers and midwives can be taught simple reflexology techniques for labour.

Post-natally, reflexology can be used to stimulate the placenta's expulsion and contraction of the uterus, and to stimulate urinary and bowel function. Receiving reflexology can relax the mother, help recovery, rebalance hormones and spinal posture and promote breastfeeding.

Progress Check

1   How might reflexology before conception help the health of mother and baby?
2   What reflexes would you consider avoiding in the first three months of pregnancy?
3   Why would you work the breast and pituitary reflexes to encourage the onset of labour?
3   What reflexes would you consider working to promote breast feeding and why?

Reflexology for clients with disability

Reflexology can be a very welcome experience for people with a disability. They can be plagued by minor symptoms to do with their disability, which when relieved can greatly enhance their well-being and self-esteem. This can have a positive effect on all their relationships. Research in Switzerland, for instance, has shown that giving reflexology to hospitalised patients with cerebral palsy reduced the occurrence of spasms, improved bladder and bowel function and sleep, and greatly improved the overall well-being of patients.

Depending on the nature and extent of the disability, where possible, teaching the client or care-giver how to do simple reflexology between treatments can help maintain the effects. Being able to give herself reflexology can give the client a degree of participation in maximising health and activity which she may otherwise be unable to have.

When giving treatments the reflexologist needs to consider each client as an individual and adapt the treatment to the particular nature and circumstances. The following may need to be considered:

- depending on disability, access to the premises and to toilet facilities
- arrangements for the client's comfort during treatment and for the practitioner's access to the feet or hands
- arrangement for permission of parent, guardian or physician where necessary
- depending on the disability, the handling of the feet or hands may need careful attention.

REMEMBER

Approach the client holistically, seeing and treating the whole person, not just the disability.

GOOD PRACTICE

Ensure good, safe access to treatment locations. Engage the client as much as possible in the treatment. Aim to improve overall health. Obtain permission of the physician, parent or guardian when necessary.

ACTIVITY

1 Listen to a series of BBC Radio 4's Tuesday night programme, *In Touch*, which is by and for disabled people.

2 Contact one of the support groups for a particular disability and ask for any free publications they produce for their members. Think about what reflexes may need attention for this particular disability.

3 Research local community support available for a particular type of disability. Make a note of these. How would you approach treating a young person with this disability compared to an elderly person?

1   What general precautions need you observe when treating clients with disability?
2   What advantages can self-treatment have for these clients?
3   What changes do you need to make to your clinic or home to ensure easier access for disabled clients?

Reflexology for clients with AIDS

For the client

Clients who are HIV-positive or have AIDS need not necessarily be treated in any way differently from other clients – that is, they are treated holistically with full respect for the healing force within them and consideration for their individual condition. Treatment can be geared to the individual circumstances but the immune and stress reflexes will naturally receive particular attention. Bear in mind that the state of mind and emotions of the client may be particularly sensitive, depending on how much they understand and accept their situation. The nature of reflexology needs to be explained to the client, with its positive contribution defined but without giving an impression of false hope; the client's co-operation and engagement in the treatment is also important. The receiving of reflexology can act as a catalyst for the client to get to know her body and work with it to maximise health and the vital force.

Reflexology can definitely help the HIV-positive client to postpone the onset of AIDS by strengthening the immune system and other body functions. Even if AIDS is present, reflexology can help the body to fight infections and probably go some way at least to relieve distressing symptoms. By providing the contact of caring human touch, reflexology can counter the tendency towards feelings of isolation which only drain the body's reserves of vitality.

For the practitioner

For the practitioner, certain precautions need to be taken. Primarily this concerns avoiding any contact with broken skin, or any situation where contact with the person's blood or bodily fluids may occur. This should not normally be a feature of reflexology anyway, but extra care needs to be taken when handling feet or hands.

GOOD PRACTICE

Keep an accepting attitude towards the client while ensuring safety for yourself.

ACTIVITY

Contact your nearest advice centre for AIDS. Ask them for an information pack about this condition and for any talks you may attend to learn more about it.

Reflexology for clients with drug dependencies

These clients benefit from the holistic care of reflexology just as others do. They are treated with the same respect and non-judgmental attitude. In fact the holistic approach through reflexology enables them to better understand themselves and their condition and helps them heal their relationship with the world in ways that are usually not included in standard treatment. Often when they learn about the nature of the vital force within them, their own self-worth as an expression of that force, how it may be hindered or helped through lifestyle, and how it may be liberated to work for them towards health through reflexology and other simple choices within their means, such knowledge fosters a positive self image and outlook that helps them to make the necessary changes. Receiving reflexology allows them to experience the benefits of human touch in a safe, non-threatening environment; this may be completely new to them. The eye contact with the practitioner, the interchange about what the feet reveal, engages the person positively with her body, re-establishes the mind-body connections, promotes integration over fragmentation and isolation – at all levels of being.

In our culture, we tend to think of 'drug addiction', or 'drug abuse' as only to do with illegal use of hashish, narcotics and related substances. We do not readily acknowledge such legal forms of drug dependency as smoking, alcohol dependency, or use of prescription drugs such as Valium, amphetamines, and Prozac. Even food can be abused as if it were a drug, when it substitutes for the 'feel good factor' or sense of self-esteem and well-being. These we normally get from basic self-acceptance and self-love which nurtures us and allows loving relationships with others. Eating disorders can be considered a kind of addiction, since the person is in effect using the food, or in some cases lack of it, as a means to a certain state of mind. As practitioners we can be alert to the possible incidence of such hidden dependency in our clients – often unacknowledged – as we conduct the case history. We can then advise the client or refer them to the appropriate counsellor or agency.

Reflexes

Whatever the drug abused, the same basic approach is taken: to regain healthy balance in the body, mind, emotions and in life habits. The practitioner also bears in mind that certain organs of the body will have been weakened by substance abuse. These include particularly the liver and kidneys. The liver works to detoxify the blood of the drug; the kidneys to balance acid and alkaline and filter the blood of remaining impurities before excretion. If smoking is the habit, the lungs will have been congested and/or weakened. Working the eliminative channel reflexes is extremely important to cleanse the body tissues of the residue of the drugs. Working the immune reflexes is very important, as is working the glands, stress and nervous system reflexes to help regain a sense of calm, and nurture the energy to throw off the addiction.

Teaching the client to work her own reflexes for a few minutes daily at intervals and whenever needed in a crisis can be an important component of treatment. When she is pulled back by the negative side effects of withdrawal, and becomes anxious, nervous and in pain, whether physical or emotional, working the reflexes can help to see her through the crisis as well as providing an alternative positive activity to taking the drug. The solar plexus and stress reflexes are particularly important here.

The practitioner gives regular treatments which create an accepting and loving environment as well as providing relief from anxiety, and a counterbalance to a negative self-image. We substitute positive therapeutic sensations for negative, imbalancing ones. At the same time as receiving treatment, the client needs advice on proper nutrition which will aid your efforts at cleansing and healing the body.

When treating clients with drug dependency, remember they may be particularly prone to unconscious transference within the therapeutic context; aware of this, the practitioner needs to keep the relationship within appropriate boundaries. Review the chapters on the therapeutic relationship and communication skills.

Watch for signs of relapse

The client needs support through the process of recovery as there are many pitfalls awaiting her. There may be times when she feels frustrated or impatient for results, feels exhausted or depressed. She may express self-pity, a tendency to blame others or expect too much from them; she seeks excuses to return to the habit. A danger point is when some considerable progress has been made and she feels she has mastered it and need no longer abstain; she may become complacent and let up on daily disciplines. She may feel she no longer needs advice and support from others, no one can tell her anything new. All these pitfalls and others await the client and set the stage for a relapse. Help the client to set a series of short-term realistic goals which can be reached with normal human effort. Drug dependency has been years in the making and it will take many years of slow steady effort to come to terms with the negative patterns that have created it and to cleanse the negative residues from the system so it can return to its natural vibrant state of health.

In addition to treating the main cleansing and toning reflexes, the practitioner must listen also to the feet and let the treatment and recommendations be adapted to the individual. Coming for treatment two, or better three times, a week is recommended with treatments lasting 20 to 30 minutes. Little-and-often is again the key.

Reflexology in itself is unlikely to bring a complete recovery. It should be part of a multi-faceted approach involving diet, counselling, visualisations, prayer or meditation, and balancing exercises such as yoga and t'ai chi.

REMEMBER
Drug dependency can be a form of escape from a negative self-image, or extremely negative experiences. Reflexology replaces negative sensations about the body with positive ones.

GOOD PRACTICE

Treat little and often. Aim treatment to relieve anxieties, cleanse the body and support the client through the difficult times.

ACTIVITY
Contact your nearest Drug Advisory Service. Ask for an information pack about drug use/abuse and, if you can, attend a talk or training on this subject.

Progress Check

1   What is often at the root of drug dependency?
2   How can a holistic understanding of the mind and body help a drug-dependent client in ways the conventional mechanistic approach cannot?
3   What precautions would you observe when treating these clients?
4   What organs are most likely to have been weakened through drug abuse?

Reflexology for the psychiatric client

All the benefits of balance, integration and inner communication which are encouraged through reflexology can greatly improve life for these clients. Here the mental and emotional aspects of treatment are to the fore; reflexology, though working primarily on the physical level, can certainly affect these. Reflexology can influence the energetic relationships between the various organs and systems and between the body and the mind. To give some examples: healthy glandular function and healthy reproductive organs can have an effect on emotions; being full of waste in the colon can affect the head and/or heart and cloud the understanding – a thorough cleanse on the physical level unblocks congestion affecting the emotional and mental sphere. Anxiety and depression can both reflect the health of the kidneys and liver and affect these organs considerably through the stress response.

Considerations about working in consultation with the client's physician and family members need to be taken into account when treating these patients; permission may need to be obtained. The effects of medications are taken into account and also the effects of reflexology treatment on the metabolism of medication. For example, the body's response may be subdued by any sedative medication the patient is on; the liver will be overburdened with detoxifying the drug residues. Yet reflexology will have its effect and careful monitoring of medication dosage is needed.

Treatment sessions should be frequent and short, with the aim being for the client to have a relaxing and positive experience within the safety of the therapeutic space. This allows the person to release defences and re-integrate.

Reflexes which may need particular attention for these patients include: diaphragm and solar plexus, glands – especially pituitary and adrenal, nervous system and stress reflexes, brain reflexes for the hypothalamus. Apply touch to both head and sacrum or solar plexus reflexes simultaneously to encourage connection between head and body, to ground any mental hyperactivity.

> **REMEMBER**
> Psychiatric clients suffer from a complex of factors. Reflexology needs to be part of a multi-angled approach. Engage the participation of the client and family members in treatment as much as possible in the individual circumstances.

GOOD PRACTICE

Obtain the co-operation of family members and physician for the treatment. Depending on the condition, it may be wise to treat in privacy but within a clinic or hospital setting, never alone.

Self-treatment with reflexology

One of the distinguishing features of reflexology is that it readily lends itself to self-treatment. Usually this is a very good idea. Teaching the client to work on certain reflexes has many advantages such as:

◆   helping her take responsibility for, and participate in, her own healing process
◆   reinforcing the work done during treatment so that the cumulative effects of reflexology are enhanced.

It is true that self-treatment is not quite as good as receiving – for one important reason: the client cannot be so totally relaxed and open to receiving. In addition, it may not be possible for the client to reach certain reflexes for one reason or another. Some people will just not take to the idea of treating themselves and this must be respected. Furthermore, it is unlikely that a person will wish to give a complete treatment to both feet. In the right circumstances, however, self-treatment is a valuable addition to professional care.

It is not a good idea to give the impression that one needs to work a tender reflex until all tenderness ceases. This might lead the client to overwork a reflex in her enthusiasm. While reflexology is highly unlikely to imbalance the body, theoretically anything taken to excess has such a potential and we must allow for completely idiosyncratic reactions.

Take time to instruct the client carefully about which reflexes to work and what is aimed at by treating each one. Provide the client with a map of the foot or hand. Demonstrate the technique and then have the client practise with your guidance before going home. Show the client the best positions for working the reflexes, and how to use the supporting hand.

Discuss with her the best times for her to work, for example in the bath, while travelling, whatever is best for the individual. Three to five minutes once or twice a day is sufficient for most people, although others find that twenty minutes of work is not too much. The practitioner needs to judge each client individually. Again little-and-often usually brings gradual, consistent results. Ask the client to keep a record of the work they do and any response they notice.

 Progress Check

1 What are the advantages of teaching a client self-treatment?
2 What are the disadvantages?
3 What advice would you give a client about how often to treat herself?
4 What advice would you give about how to treat tender reflexes?

Reflexology in hospitals

Many hospitals are more open to complementary medicine practitioners either in a voluntary capacity or employed as staff than they were a few years ago. There the caring therapeutic touch reflexology gives is specially welcome and supports and enhances the healing processes of the body. Patients welcome it because reflexology aims to treat the person, not the illness, and all too often this point of view is lacking in hospitals where the focus is on controlling the disease itself. Staff receive an indirect benefit because patients will be much more comfortable, much less demanding. Reflexology lends itself readily to the hospital setting. It requires no special equipment or even furniture. Being so adaptable, it can be given with the client seated, in bed or even standing if necessary, and if the feet cannot be treated the hands certainly can.

Reflexology can be used in a variety of conditions and situations within the hospital. For example, we have mentioned using it for peri-natal care. It can be used after surgery to help speed the healing of the wound and allay the shock the body has experienced. It is ideal as an augmentation to physiotherapy. Patients in care for psychiatric or drug dependency problems can receive benefit as described above. Reflexology may be especially appreciated in the hospice setting. Again the caring therapeutic touch gives needed comfort and helps relieve some minor symptoms of terminal illness.

> **REMEMBER**
> Even within a busy, noisy hospital setting, try to create the atmosphere of the therapeutic space: a peaceful calm, a sense of security that allows the body and mind of the patient to relax deeply, release tensions and worries for a few moments – freeing the vital force to heal.

When working in wards within hospitals, try to ensure the maximum privacy possible in the circumstances. If it is suitable and desired by the patient, teach some simple reflexology to her or a family member or friend. Do not aim to give a long treatment, especially in the first stages. Always treat both feet and try to touch the major areas of both but it is not necessary to treat every single reflex. The aim is to raise the overall health of the body rather than work specific reflexes relating to the condition. Be aware that the feet or hands may be extra sensitive, especially in areas related to the site of trauma or surgery and only a very light touch is needed. Sometimes just touching a reflex for a sustained period of time, allowing the energy to begin to circulate to and from the point, until the point becomes warmer, is enough treatment. Remember to use the cross reflexes, if indicated, to re-reinforce or replace treatment to other parts.

ACTIVITY

Write a letter to the nurse in charge of a hospital ward or service. Explain clearly what reflexology entails and its aims. Describe its benefits for the patients and staff on a particular ward. Offer to give a talk and demonstration to the nursing staff. If desired, volunteer to come on a regular basis for a defined period of time to try out reflexology in a hospital setting.

Progress Check

1 What are some advantages of reflexology for patients in hospital?
2 What are some disadvantages of giving treatment in hospital as opposed to treating in a clinic or home setting?
3 What is the aim of the treatment when treating in hospital?
4 Why is it important to engage the interest and co-operation of the staff when treating in hospital?

Care in the community

A holistic approach to care recognises that our health is constantly influenced by the world around us. Reflexologists cannot provide every aspect of care and support. Often we recognise that a client may need special support with a particular problem beyond our scope or knowledge. We may have a client whose health is being affected significantly by social, financial, personal or other problems and these need outside help. It is very beneficial then for the reflexologist to be aware of some of the major support services in the area, either local or national ones.

There are local organisations and also local branches of national organisations. Some support is also supplied by social services departments of local councils.

ACTIVITY

1 Use the Yellow Pages or a local directory, library, or contact the Citizens Advice Bureau or local council and social services or your medical centre to find out about the services provided by the following organisations. Make a note of the telephone numbers and addresses:

WRVS   RELATE   Cruse   Arthritis Care   National Asthma Campaign   Alcoholics Anonymous   Samaritans

2 Match the following organisations with the services they provide:

Rape Crisis Centre	Home help, day care centres, etc.
MIND	Voluntary work, gardening, decorating
AIDS helpline	District Nurse will call to check on health
Age Concern	Helps with mental health concerns
Royal National Institute for the Blind	Support for elderly persons' needs
Social Services	Help in cases of rape or sexual abuse
Youth Groups, Scouts, Guides	Provides advice and practical help for the partially sighted

Key Terms

You need to know what these terms mean. Go back through the chapter or check in the glossary to find out.

- Self-esteem
- Post-natal
- AIDS
- Transference
- Peri-natal
- HIV-positive
- Hospice
- Relapse

HAND REFLEXOLOGY

After working through this chapter you will be able to:

♦ understand the structure of the hands
♦ understand the differences between the hands and feet as regards reflexology
♦ understand the practical advantages of working the hands instead of the feet
♦ understand some of the practical adaptations and techniques to use when working the hands.

Although reflexology is most widely known as a 'foot treatment', its efficacy is also well proven when reflexes of the hands are stimulated. The hands are anatomically related to and very much like the feet, but there are also important differences.

Giving to the giver

Giving reflexology treatment to the hands is an effective alternative to treating the feet. If we stop to think about it, they *are* usually associated with doing and giving. So it's nice for them to be still and receive care from another person. Also, as we have seen in the introduction, the fingers and thumbs of the hands are among the three most sensitive areas of the body. Sensory pathways from these areas especially stimulate the brain, providing deep sensations of well-being. The hands have their own special quality.

Structure of the hands

There are eight small carpal bones in the wrist arranged in two rows of four bones each. These bones are named: scaphoid, lunate, triquetral, pisiform, trapezium, trapezoid, capitate and hamate. There are five metacarpal bones and fourteen phalanges on the hand, two in the pollex or thumb, and three in each of the other fingers.

The major muscles of the hand are on the palmar aspect and include: the thenar eminence and hypothenar eminence, the tendon of the thumb flexor, the tendons of the four finger flexors and the tendon of the palmaris, the flexor retinaculum and the palmar aponeurosis.

On the dorsal aspect there are the superficial flexors of the fingers extending from the superficial muscles of the forearm.

Advantages of using the hands for reflexology

Working the hands has several practical advantages. It can be used in situations in which foot reflexology is not possible. Some people may be so embarrassed about letting their feet be touched that they will not allow them to be exposed for treatment, but they will be comfortable with a hand treatment. In some instances it may not be possible to reach the feet but access to the hands is available. For example, it is possible to give hand reflexology in a semi-public place such as a workplace setting, while travelling or at a bedside in a hospital ward. In other circumstances it may be that a foot has been injured or a client is suffering from skin complaints which make using the hands preferable. I once had a student who had lost one foot in an accident, but treatment was still possible on the hand. In all these instances hand reflexology can be substituted.

Treating the hands may have particular advantage for those hard of hearing, as verbal communication will be enhanced by the close proximity. We can all remember how comforting it is for a loved one to hold our hand; this memory is surely stimulated by reflexology,

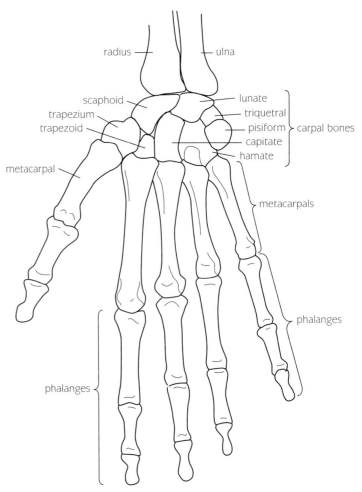

Fig. 10.1 *The bones of the wrist and hand (dorsal view)*

GOOD PRACTICE

Use a lighter pressure when working the hands of the elderly or children.

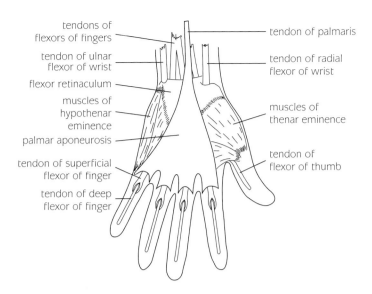

tendons of
flexors of fingers

tendon of ulnar
flexor of wrist

flexor retinaculum

muscles of
hypothenar
eminence

palmar aponeurosis

tendon of superficial
flexor of finger

tendon of deep
flexor of finger

tendon of palmaris

tendon of radial
flexor of wrist

muscles of
thenar eminence

tendon of
flexor of thumb

Fig. 10.2 *(a) The muscles of the hand, palmar view*

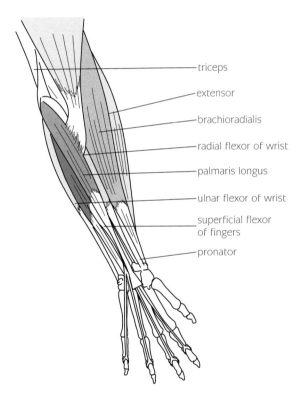

triceps

extensor

brachioradialis

radial flexor of wrist

palmaris longus

ulnar flexor of wrist

superficial flexor
of fingers

pronator

Fig. 10.2 *(b) Superficial muscles of the forearm*

enhancing the effect of security and loving care. Sometimes, in highly
emotional states, the hands are the most immediately accessible and
acceptable point of contact when others would be rejected. For some
people receiving treatment on the hands is very powerful if they are
usually using their hands to give of themselves to others.

However, some clients may at first find it even more difficult to 'let go'
and completely relax the hand and arm than they do when receiving
treatment on the foot. The practitioner needs to gently coax the client to
relax and allow the arm to be loose and receptive. This may take some
time, but repeated reminders and reassurance will bring results.

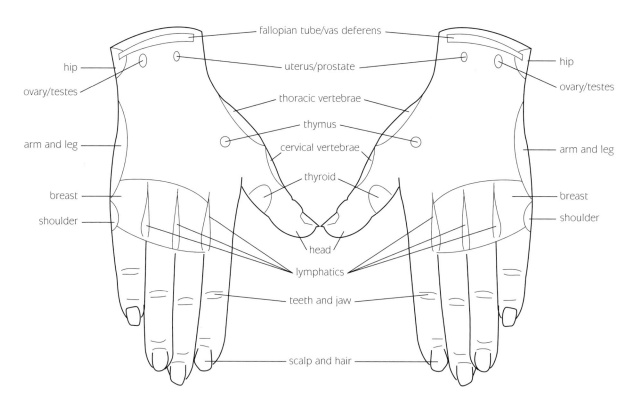

Fig. 10.3 *(a) A map of the reflexes of the hand, dorsal view (courtesy of Kristine Walker)*

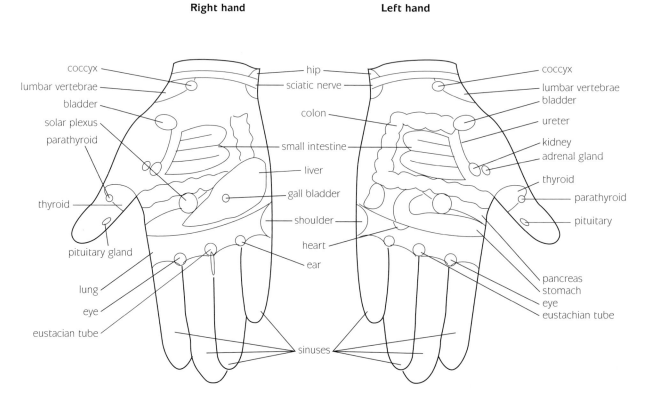

Fig. 10.3 *(b) A map of the reflexes of the hand, palmar view (courtesy of Kristine Walker)*

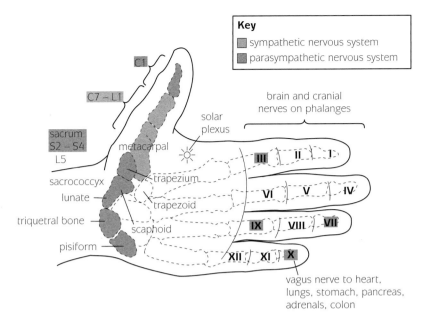

Fig. 10.3 *(c) The cranial nerves and autonomic nervous system in the hand*
Additional material courtesy of Association Reflex Therapy Total Faure-Alderson

Self-reflexology on the hands

Teaching clients to work their reflexes on their hands instead of the feet may be better for some. Hands are easier to get to and it is easier to treat your own hands than your feet. This fact may be especially important for someone who is for any reason less mobile and flexible in their range of movement. Hands may be worked without anyone else noticing, so treatment can be given little-and-often in almost any setting.

Here are two examples of techniques which can be taught to clients for self-reflexology:

- A dynamic holding, using either light or deeper pressure, with a finger or finger/thumb either side of the webbed area between the thumb and index finger, relating to the bronchioles can be very effective in treating coughs.
- A dragging pressure applied along each of the five metacarpal grooves up to the base of the fingers, with the thumb on the palmar side and index finger on the dorsal has been found to help regulate blood pressure. This should be repeated for 15–20 minutes on each hand several times a day.

Practicalities when working the hands

In general, the same considerations and precautions for treating the hands exist as for treating the feet, with the client's comfort the primary consideration. The same care should be taken to create a therapeutic space, no matter what the actual venue. The state of mind of the giver is again an important factor.

The same basic thumb and finger walking techniques, hook-in-back-up, pivot-on-a-point, light holding, breathing-with-pressure can be used as in foot reflexology. It is always best to give a full treatment using a sequence such as the one suggested in Chapter 7 – always beginning and ending with relaxation. But if time is limited, working the relaxation reflexes, the glands and any symptom site reflex would be a good approach. Again, use one hand to support the client's hand while the other works the reflexes.

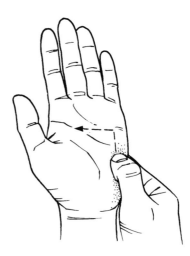

Fig. 10.4 *Thumb walking across the colon in zone 5*

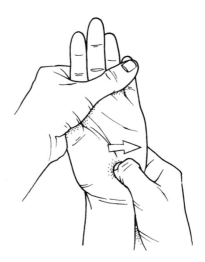

Fig. 10.5 *Hook-in-back-up on the sigmoid colon area*

When treating the hand the practitioner may be seated either beside or facing the client, depending on the situation and what is most comfortable for both. As when treating the feet the practitioner's hands should be washed before and after treatment. A thick towel may be used if necessary to keep the hands warm. A small pillow may be useful for supporting the client's arm and hand.

When treating the hand the practitioner will be in closer proximity to the client's face than when working on the feet so care may be necessary to avoid 'invading' the client's space in an unwelcome way. On the other hand, some clients appreciate the closer contact; and some, for example the hard of hearing, may need this proximity.

Differences between hands and feet

Bear in mind that the reflexes on the hand are distributed slightly differently than on the feet. The chest and abdominal region of the major organs is much more compressed. This means that the reflexes will be deeper and possibly harder to contact. At the same time, the head-neck-throat area on the thumb and fingers is much greater and easier to reach. Again we find that these are the areas with greatest reflex stimulation to the cerebral cortex. It may be that, for this reason, these reflexes should in fact be worked on the hands rather than the feet; as they are more easily stimulated so treatment may be more effective.

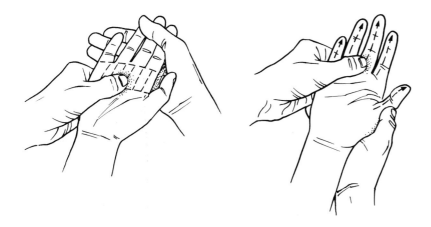

Fig. 10.6 *(a) Working the chest area (b) Working the fingers for the head area reflexes*

Some reflexologists find that it is sometimes preferable to include work on the hands even if the feet are receiving treatment. For example, if they feel some blockage to progress in a course of treatments and they switch from working the feet to working the hands, the blockage is overcome more quickly than might otherwise have been the case.

Another difference is that generally when working the hands we reserve the thumb for working the palm and sides of the hands where the tissues are thicker and the index finger for working the dorsal aspect.

Some reflexologists feel that the hands are not as sensitive as the feet because they are not as protected. Hence tender areas may not register as easily. However, this may result more from individual differences, as some people's hands may be just as sensitive as their feet. For this reason, it may be that such individuals actually need some reflexes to be worked on the hands rather than the feet as they are more easily stimulated, thus making their treatment more effective.

Kristine Walker, who has made a special study of hand reflexology, gives the following advice for treating some specific points.

1   Use the knuckle of the thumb or index finger to treat the pituitary reflex.

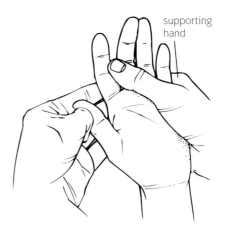

Fig. 10.7 *Working the pituitary reflex on the thumb, using the knuckle of the thumb*

2   To work the shoulder, elbow, arm and knee-hip reflexes, work the fifth metacarpal and carpal bones of the lateral palm and wrist. To work, sandwich the client's palm between your own two palms. When working on your client's right hand, your left hand should be on top, and vice versa. Allow the client's little finger to rest in the web between your left thumb and index finger. Your right thumb can now work down the side of the hand to locate the reflexes:

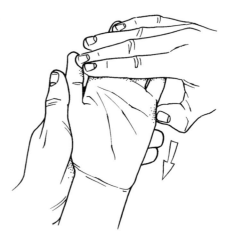

Fig. 10.8 *Working the shoulder and upper arm*

3   For the upper lymphatic reflexes, work down the dorsal grooves between the metacarpals using the index finger with the thumb on the palm for support.

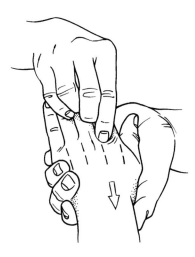

Fig. 10.9 *Working the lymphatic reflexes in the chest*

ACTIVITY

Practise working the head and toe, then the chest-lung reflexes on a partner. Think about the differences or similarities as you experience them and discuss these with your partner. Then ask your partner for feedback on any differences or similarities she may have felt. Reverse your roles so you may experience treatment on both feet and hands. Again discuss. Compare notes with any other students in your group.

Progress Check

1 What are some differences between the anatomy of the foot and of the hand?
2 What are three advantages to working on the hands?
3 Why might the hands be more sensitive than the feet? not so sensitive?
4 Why are hands particularly suited to self-treatment?

Key Terms

You need to know what these terms mean. Go back through the chapter or check in the glossary to find out.

- Carpal bones
- Palmar aspect
- Pollex

11 LIFESTYLE ADVICE TO THE REFLEXOLOGY CLIENT

After working through this chapter you will be able to:

♦ appreciate the value of giving some guidance to clients in areas that will positively affect their health and support your reflexology treatments

♦ understand the importance of good nutrition as the basis of long term positive health

♦ recognise the body's basic nutritional requirements

♦ have a basic understanding of some therapeutic diets that support reflexology objectives

♦ understand the importance of relaxation for the body's optimum functioning and of using basic relaxation techniques for yourself as well as your clients

♦ understand the role of exercise in relation to positive health.

Any holistic approach to health care involves attention to those aspects of our lives which each of us can undertake to make as healthy as possible. These include, as a minimum, the areas of nutrition, exercise and relaxation. As reflexologists we are concerned to help clients maintain their health beyond the course of treatments, so we naturally have an interest in seeing our clients make improvements in these aspects of their lives. However, we must first educate ourselves in the basics of a healthy lifestyle so we can advise clients appropriately or know when to refer them to other qualified practitioners.

Diet and nutrition

A reflexologist is in a position to offer sound advice to clients about changes in their diet which will support what she is trying to achieve with reflexology. To this end some basic information and ideas are offered here. If a serious deficiency or problem related to diet is present, referral should be made to a practitioner with the relevant expertise, such as a nutritionist or physician.

'We are what we eat'

As holistic practitioners, reflexologists have long pointed out that the average western diet is harmful to health and in fact lays the foundation for many diseases. They have realised that the cumulative effect of years on a denatured diet can amount to stress on the body's processes, and can gradually weaken organs, or create blood which is excessively acid or imbalanced in its composition. A denatured diet contains a high proportion of processed or refined food products, often with harmful additives, or which are produced in such a way as to adversely affect the body's health. For example, chemical herbicides and pesticides used to produce foods can leave toxic residues in the body; the hormones and antibiotics used in the production of meat and dairy products can build up in the body and affect its healthy functioning.

> **REMEMBER**
> Food is medicine and medicine is food.

Refined foods are lacking in fibre content which, while not in itself an essential nutrient, plays an important role in maintaining health. Lack of fibre has been implicated in such diseases as cancer of the colon, diverticulitis, obesity, ischaemic heart disease as well as in gallstones, constipation and haemorrhoids. Fibre helps the body evacuate its waste through the colon. By holding water it softens the stool and by increasing its bulk, it speeds the transit time of faeces through the colon.

The basic nutrients

All of our food ultimately comes from plants, and secondhand from animals. Our daily intake of food supplies us with the following nutrients essential for life and health: carbohydrates, fats, proteins, minerals, vitamins.

Carbohydrates

These provide the body's primary source of energy and are made of three basic elements: carbon, hydrogen and oxygen. Carbohydrates are sugars which are converted by the body into fuel, enabling it to perform its many functions. Sugars come in three forms:

- simple or mono-saccharides (such as fructose and galactose)
- disaccharides or pairs of sugars linked together (such as lactose, and sucrose)
- complex carbohydrates or chains of hundreds of simple sugars.

The first two are soluble in water and taken up quickly by the body. Complex carbohydrates are not water soluble and are broken down and absorbed slowly so that their fuel is provided slowly and steadily.

Fats

Like carbohydrates, fats are made of carbon, hydrogen and oxygen and provide a highly concentrated source of energy which can be stored and used instead of carbohydrates when necessary. They also contain essential fatty acids needed by every cell. Fats are a combination of glycerol and fatty acids in three forms: saturated, monosaturated and polyunsaturated. A high consumption of saturated fatty acids is recognised to be a factor in hypertension and heart disease, while polyunsaturated fats supply the needed nutrients without causing such problems.

Proteins

Proteins are complex substances made of amino acids but also containing nitrogen, sulphur, iron, and other minerals in small amounts. When protein is eaten, the molecule is broken down into its individual amino acids which are used by the body's cells for their metabolic functions. For example: growth and repair of tissues, production of enzymes, regulating the balance of water and acidity, the formation of antibodies. When absolutely necessary, the body will burn proteins for fuel.

Minerals

About 60 different minerals have been identified in the body, of which 21 are considered to be essential. An essential mineral is one that must be supplied in the food; it cannot be manufactured in the body. It also performs a function necessary to life, for example, regulating metabolic processes and building tissue. Some minerals are required in substantial amounts, others in minute or trace amounts. Three minerals tend to be low among western peoples: calcium, zinc and iron. The chart shows some of the important minerals, their functions in the body, and their signs of deficiency.

	Calcium Ca	Chromium Cr	Copper Cu	Germanium Ge	Iron Fe

Main functions	bones
	teeth
	muscle
	  contraction
	co-enzymes
	blood clotting
		carbohydrate
		  metabolism
		insulin
		  production
			haemoglobin
			  factor
			co-enzymes
			nerve function
					haemoglobin
					other
					  enzymes

Signs of deficiency	irritability
	muscle cramps
	fractures
	bowlegs
	air swallowing
		glucose-
		  intolerance
					bluish film
					  over eyeball
					pale mucous
					  membranes

Factors which increase requirements	pregnancy
	breastfeeding
	growth
		exposure to
		  chemicals
				diarrhoea
				use of diuretics
				use of aspirin
				use of
				  corticosteroids
					excessive
					  blood loss
					  (menstruation,
					  wounds,
					  injury)
					diarrhoea
					pregnancy/
					  lactation

Deficiency caused by consumption of	**diet high in**
	proteins
	phosphorus ,
	  (cola drinks,
	  meat)
	diet low in
	dairy products
		diet high in
		refined sugars
		
		diet low in
		cereals
		brewer's yeast
			diet high in
			zinc
			molybdenum
			iron
			diet low in
			liver
			cereals
			leafy
			  vegetables
			almonds
			seafood
				diet high in
				
				diet low in
				beans
				tuna fish
				oysters
				garlic
					diet high in
					coffee
					zinc
					cadmium
					diet low in
					oysters
					meat

Illnesses associated with deficiency	rickets		Menke's kinky
			  hair syndrome
			aneurysms
			cerebral
			  degeneration
					iron-def.
					anaemia

High-risk groups	pregnant
	lactating
	children
	the elderly
	  (particularly
	  women)
		sweet eaters
		alcohol
		  consumers
		the elderly
			–	people with
				  lowered
				  immunity
					women
					pregnancy/
					  lactation

Vitamins

The word vitamin was coined by a Polish chemist, Casimir Funk in 1922 to name a crystalline nitrogen-containing substance (amine) which he had isolated and found to cure beri-beri. He identified this and subsequent such substances as 'vita – amines' or amines essential to life; the e was later dropped to give our word 'vitamin' when it was found that not all vitamins contained nitrogen. Like the trace minerals, the quantities of vitamins present in foods and the amounts we need are minute compared with the 'macro' nutrients: proteins, carbohydrates, fats and minerals.

	Magnesium Mg	Manganese Mn	Molybdenum Mo	Potassium K	Selenium Se	Zinc Zn
Main functions	energy generation muscle contraction nerve function vitamin co-factor bones and teeth	cartilage production antioxidant energy generation	involved in metabolism of uric acid, aldehydes, sulphites	cellular balance nerve function muscle function	antioxidant enzyme co-factor	hormone synthesis vitamin A co-factor nucleic acid production antioxidant immune function
Signs of deficiency	muscle cramps nervousness			weak reflexes		loss of smell/taste white spots on nails
Factors which increase require-ments	stress pregnancy/ lactation diarrhoea use of the 'pill' use of diuretics		air pollution (SO_2) Crohn's disease		air pollution (SO_2) heavy metals	stress injury/ wounds use of the 'pill' use of cortico-steroids pregnancy/ lactation
Deficiency caused by consumption of	diet high in alcohol calcium phosphorus	diet high in calcium phosphorus potassium	diet high in copper proteins sulphite	diet high in salt coffee black tea cocoa refined sugar	diet high in zinc sulphur	diet high in alcohol copper calcium cadmium lead
	diet low in nuts, almonds seafood leafy vegetables figs	diet low in black tea cereals seeds leafy vegetables	diet low in cabbage, esp cauliflower beans carrots	diet low in bananas potatoes vegetables fruit cereals	diet low in liver brewer's yeast seafood wholewheat bread	diet low in oysters eggs
Illnesses associated with deficiency	convulsions	infertility bony abnormalities	neurological abnormalities bony abnormalities impotence	infertility renal hypertrophy paralysis	hepatic necrosis muscular dystrophy	dwarfism infertility
High-risk groups	alcohol consumers diabetics pregnant/ lactating the elderly		children	drug consumers elderly	the entire population	pregnancy/ lactation children drinkers, alcohol consumers the elderly

Vitamins are divided into the water-soluble (vitamins C and the B complex group) and fat-soluble groups (vitamins A, D, E). The amount of each vitamin needed ranges widely – we need 10,000 times more vitamin C than B12 for example – yet a deficiency of any vitamin is a serious matter. A deficiency can induce specific clinical symptoms which are cleared up when the vitamin is supplied. The enzymes needed for transforming our food into a form useful for our tissues are to a large extent dependent on co-enzyme factors to be able to do their job. Co-enzymes are usually vitamins. The presence of other substances in our food or diet influences the absorption and availability of vitamins in our bodies.

Water and air

In addition to nutrients from foods, our bodies also need adequate amounts of good quality water and air. Unfortunately, in our modern world the quality of both of these substances is also often compromised or poor because of pollution and other factors. It can also be the case that we don't actually take enough water or air due to our habits and lifestyle. For example, it has been shown in the US that in 1994, the population actually consumed on average more soft drinks than water for the first time. If we don't allow ourselves adequate exercise and rest we may not be breathing deeply at any time during the day. This in turn will affect the amount of oxygen that our body takes in.

Progress Check

1 What are the basic nutritional requirements of the human body?
2 What role does fibre play in the body's health?
3 What are the fat soluble vitamins?
4 What is the role of proteins in the diet?
5 How can lack of adequate amounts and quality of air and water affect health?

ACTIVITY

Research and prepare a table, like the one on minerals on pages 176–77, in which you organise information on vitamins. For each vitamin give its function, signs of deficiency, good quality food sources, factors which may deplete it (such as refined sugars, pregnancy, loss of blood, etc.), and substances necessary for its optimum metabolism.

Healthful diets

If ingesting certain foods lays the foundation for disease, then avoiding them and replacing them with fresh foods full of life allows the body the chance to alter this foundation and hence allows recovery and healing to take place. Such a change may be termed a therapeutic cleansing diet. Basically, foods which have a negative effect on the body when consumed in too great a quantity are avoided or left out altogether. They include the following:

- all fried foods
- meat and eggs

- white bread, cakes, biscuits and processed flour products
- sugar, especially white, refined
- chocolate
- salt
- refined oils
- synthetic food additives.

In addition some people find that some of the following foods provoke allergic reactions or sensitivity. These foods include: gluten from certain grains, especially wheat; cow's milk and milk-derived products (goat's milk may be tolerated); chocolate, shellfish, nuts, strawberries, eggs, coffee, tomatoes, alcohol.

It is generally recommended that cheese and dairy products are eliminated in a cleansing diet, especially hard cheeses. Milk products are thought to be 'cold' and somewhat heavy in nature and harder to digest, so stimulating the over-production of mucus which is very clogging to the system. If they are consumed they should be taken warmed and blended with warming spices such as cinnamon, pepper, cardamom, allspice, a traditional way, in fact, of preparing many milk-based dishes.

The therapeutic cleansing diet

Going on a therapeutic cleansing diet involves avoiding these foods at least for a certain period of time, for example three weeks. This gives the body a chance to catch up on its house cleaning and rid itself of the backlog of residues in the tissues which such a diet has created.

Cleansing involves more than just giving up certain foods. The emphasis is really not on abstaining so much as on substituting positive, life-enhancing fresh foods for negative foods which deplete our vital energy. Such foods are fresh fruits and vegetables, vegetable proteins from lentils, nuts and grains, and complex carbohydrates from vegetables and grains, i.e. root vegetables and wholegrain cereals. Sprouting grains and lentils greatly increases their vitamin content. Suggest that your clients substitute more of such foods in their diets while leaving off the foods to be avoided – gradually if necessary; there's no need for undue pressure or rigidity. Tell them they can eat as much as they wish of these foods.

We all enjoy a sweet taste but it can be found in fruits, dried fruits and dates, and in complex carbohydrates such as pasta, wholewheat bread, rice, millet and oats – for example, an oatbar is preferable to a chocolate bar. Rather than giving a sugar surge to the system, complex carbohydrates are broken down gradually, giving time-released energy which sustains and does not 'wear out' the pancreas. This is also incidentally the best way to lose weight.

Usually by the end of the cleansing period, the person's body has become so much more into balance that poor quality foods which used to be liked or craved are no longer appealing. Many people like to repeat the cleansing diet at intervals in the year as part of health maintenance. After all we clean our cars and our houses regularly, why not our bodies? Such a cleansing diet will support reflexology treatment aimed at activating the eliminative channels and clearing the build-up of toxicity or congestion in the body.

In addition we may need to advise clients to stop or cut down drinking tea and coffee. Substitute herb teas, coffee substitutes such as roasted chicory or dandelion root – or simply water instead. We all need to drink more fresh water daily: 6–8 cups.

The cleansing diet is most called for in people who you find are quite congested. Perhaps they have been constipated for years, or they find they produce a lot of phlegm or mucus, or tend to retain weight or water. It can also be used for people who have allergies, not just allergies to foods, but hay fever and skin complaints. Because it cleanses the tissues and rebalances the body, along with reflexology treatments, the body's normal response to its environment is re-established.

Liver-cleansing diet

This regime stimulates the release of wastes from the body and, in particular, clears, opens and cools the liver. It increases the flow of bile and overall liver function. It has a blood purifying effect.

For best results, follow this cleansing regime for ten days. It can be repeated after three days. Some people like to follow it in the spring and autumn particularly.

You will need daily:

Juice of one grapefruit or several oranges (3–4)
4–6 tablespoons fresh lemon or lime juice
1–3 tablespoons extra virgin olive oil
1–3 cloves crushed garlic

Mix together in a blender or by hand. Drink first thing in the morning. Follow this with hot liver-cleansing tea.

Liver-cleansing tea
Equal parts licorice root
Fenugreek seeds
Anise
Flax seed
Fennel seed
Peppermint leaves

(All can be powdered for convenience if preferred.) Steep these herbs in 700 ml (1¼ pint) hot water. You can simmer a slice of fresh ginger root in the water first for three minutes, then add the herbs and steep for 10 minutes.

During the day, continue to drink as many cups of the tea as desired. You may add honey to these other cups.

Either, eat no breakfast, or wait one hour before eating a millet or oat porridge. Having no breakfast increases the cleansing action but may not be appropriate for some people.

For lunch and dinner eat leafy vegetables, lightly steamed, in soups or raw. Eat baked potatoes or squash and as much sprouted seeds and grains as possible: alfalfa, mung bean and any others.

Snacks and desserts should be fresh fruit and nuts, in season if possible.

For best results combine this with a general cleansing diet – avoiding all meat, fish, eggs and dairy products, salt and sugar – during the ten days.

GOOD PRACTICE

Try out a cleansing diet such as that outlined above on yourself for three weeks first before you recommend it to your clients. This way you will be able to speak with authority based on personal experience of the effects.

Building diet

A cleansing diet is not suitable for everyone. For those who are weak, thin and emaciated a different approach is taken, one which tones the tissues, while not at the same time creating blockages. Such patients benefit from taking their foods warm and cooked, avoiding salads and raw foods, and eating a higher proportion of protein-rich foods and complex carbohydrates. Thick soups and gruels made with grains and lentils are recommended. Cooking with warming herbs and spices is also important to ensure thorough digestion and assimilation.

Kitcheree

This food combination comes from India where it is used in many chronic conditions, and at regular intervals for helping to tone and balance the body. It provides essential nutrition, while being light and eliminative. It cleanses the blood and tones the kidneys. It is useful as a cleansing fast food and also for debilitating conditions such as ME, anorexia and recovery from any exhausting illness.

1 cup brown or white basmati rice
½ cup mung beans or mung dahl
1 tablespoon ghee or cold pressed vegetable oil
2 pinches turmeric (or more to taste)
¼ teaspoon black mustard seed
¼ teaspoon cumin seed
6 cups water
Fresh coriander, grated coconut or parsley

Wash the rice and beans, then soak together overnight. Next day, warm the ghee or oil in a pan, add the spices and when the seeds start to 'crack', add the rice, beans and water. Stir, bring to the boil then reduce to a low temperature and cook until tender. The mixture will be a bit mushy. Add the coriander, coconut or parsley. Season with freshly ground black pepper, no salt.

Assimilation

Good digestion is as important as the quality of the food taken. Reflexology can help here by ensuring that the digestive processes are working in a balanced way. This way the vitamins, minerals and other nutrients we need from foods can be assimilated from the digestive process.

Advise clients to cook with warming carminative herbs and spices: rosemary, garlic, ginger, thyme, black pepper, cinnamon. These render food more digestible. Many people find that taking cider vinegar and honey in hot water every morning before breakfast improves digestion and assimilation and reduces excess acidity in the system.

Balancing the body through diet

One of the best approaches to an overall balanced diet for vital health is one based on a balance of alkaline and acid foods. The body is about 80% alkaline and 20% acid and the idea is to eat in such a way as to support this natural balanced ratio. This is the basis of the diet devised by Dr Hay which has been so effective for many people suffering from allergies and digestive problems, although he did not originate the concept. Following on from this is the idea that starches and proteins should not be combined in the same meal because different digestive enzymes and processes are needed to break down the different types of foods, and eating them together leads to poorer digestion and therefore weaker assimilation and more waste to be removed. Certain food groups are beneficial combinations and certain others are less beneficial and even harmful in the long run. Eating according to this diet enhances good digestion and assimilation and produces less toxic waste in the system.

One interesting fact about this diet is that it is inherently more of a vegetarian diet. Animal products are themselves acid forming and this diet keeps their consumption at a lower level, which is more conducive to health. Vegetarians naturally already eat in a more balanced alkaline-acid way. However, their diets can suffer by being overly alkaline and too light.

Eating our emotions

The quality of our mental-emotional outlook at the time of preparing and eating food definitely has its effect. We all instinctively feel that we are not hungry when we are upset. Yet too many of us will eat when we are not calm – just out of habit. This is literally eating our emotions along with our foods. Even medical science recognises the relationship between stomach ulcers and emotional states. Taking just two or three minutes to centre ourselves before meals can make all the difference. If you feel a client is not approaching meals with a positive frame of mind, simply advising her to practise the breathing techniques used at the end of the reflexology session can make a difference.

Supplements

While it is best to receive our vitamins and minerals from fresh foods, there are times when supplements may be needed. It is also true that even fresh foods may be denatured due to modern growing methods. Supplements work best when they are sourced from concentrated foods or herbs, preferably organic, and which are chelated to ensure assimilation. Kelp is an example of a superior supplement for mineral needs. There are times when the body needs an extra helping of vitamins and minerals, such as vitamins C and B6 during times of stress or acute ailments, iron when blood has been lost as during heavy periods, calcium during pregnancy and especially as we age.

REMEMBER

Whatever the therapeutic diet chosen, rigidity and fanaticism are not conducive to good health. It is the way we eat for 90% of the time that forms the foundation of our health. Occasional variations and special occasion meals will not imbalance us too far because the foundation is so strong.

Progress Check

1 Describe how eating while emotionally upset can affect health.
2 How might feeling stressed when eating affect digestion?
3 Which foods are best for enhancing life and health?
4 What is the thinking behind the Hay diet?

Exercise

This is another area in which common-sense advice given by the reflexologist can help a person improve her standard of health. Regular brisk exercise – even for just 20 or 30 minutes a day – has a very positive effect on the mind, body and emotions. Any advice given will be adjusted to the individual's age, level of fitness and personal inclinations. Clients you assess as not taking adequate exercise can be advised to begin with brisk walking until the heart begins to beat a bit harder with the effort – for about 20 minutes – no more is necessarily needed as long as it is done regularly. Some clients benefit from a class in a certain sport or type of exercise; others like to work on their own. Common sense will help you suggest a type of exercise that balances your client's current imbalances. More sedentary types benefit from regular and quite stimulating exercise while nervous active types need regular exercise and especially rhythmic, flowing types of movement. 'Workaholics', who are usually competitive, may need to find a type of exercise that involves less competition and more co-operation, such as a team sport. Dancing and swimming are excellent forms of exercise.

REMEMBER
Balance out-put with in-put so as not to deplete energy.

Exercising through yoga, qi gong or t'ai chi has some advantages over our western forms of exercise. The fundamental aim of these systems is to integrate the mind, body and spirit. They automatically include vigorous stimulating movements, along with toning and stretching ones so that all aspects of the physical body are kept fit. In addition they also include slow movements and relaxation positions, co-ordinated with breathing, which allow the body-mind to come to a level of inner peace. For this reason, they can be very helpful for those suffering from any stress or disorder in their lives.

Relaxation

Holistic medicine recognises the need for balance in all life processes. Throughout the book we have mentioned the importance of relaxation to health, as part of a healthy balance of life experiences. There are times to be active, extroverted, expending energy and there are times to be restful, introverted, conserving and restoring energy. Unfortunately a balance between these two is often lacking in our lives. We may 'collapse', slumping into a chair in front of the television in the evening, but this is not the same as positive relaxation. Our senses are constantly stimulated by foods, drugs, television, radio, work demands so that we tend to become dominated or overstimulated in the sympathetic nervous system, preventing the parasympathetic system from having its chance to work for us. Sleep, which is the most important period of relaxation, is often disturbed, or too short. Important bodily processes such as repair of tissues, full breathing and regular heartbeat occur when we are at rest.

GOOD PRACTICE

Practise relaxation and breathing techniques regularly to keep yourself 'in shape' for giving reflexology.

The body knows how to relax but most people with today's lifestyles have forgotten what it means to be truly, deeply relaxed. However there are many relaxation techniques which can be used to 're-learn' this state. The techniques need to be practised regularly for a while so that they become a new habit of mind, and the state fully experienced so it can be recognised and recalled at will. Teaching these techniques to your clients gives them the tools to take control of their lives and not be 'victims' of stress. They are particularly helpful for clients with disturbed sleep, excessive worry, depression, excessive workloads, or who are 'workaholics'; but they benefit anyone going through a particularly stressful time. They are useful for you, the practitioner, as well, by helping you through a busy day and helping you to recharge your energies and keep centred.

1 Which aspect of the nervous system is responsible for relaxation, rest and repair?
2 How can deep abdominal breathing affect the nervous system?
3 Why is it necessary to practise relaxation techniques before we can get their full benefit?

Meridians, chakras, marma, polarity

Understanding of the nature and pattern of energy flow in the body is an ancient science. Early reflexologists recognised the similarities between zone therapy and such systems as Chinese medicine, with its meridians accessed by acupuncture or acupressure (shiatsu), and Indian medicine (Ayurveda) with its marma points and yoga's chakras, the special points of energy manifestation which can be accessed by touch. Polarity therapy also uses body points including those on the feet for working with energy in a system largely derived from Ayurveda. Many practitioners like to practise reflexology within the framework of one of these medical systems because they already embrace and relate all aspects of life: diet, exercise, recreation, work, mental-emotional, even spiritual aspects of our being.

Reflexology is part of the larger tradition of Western natural medicine which, since the time of Hippocrates and Galen, has also worked holistically, relating the individual to the larger context of society, psychology and natural environment, and using the healing energy of nature, the vital force.

Key Terms

You need to know what these terms mean. Go back through the chapter or check in the glossary to find out.

- Denatured diet
- Carbohydrates
- Fats
- Proteins
- Therapeutic diet
- Minerals
- Vitamins
- Co-enzymes

Further reading

Diet and nutrition:

Ballantine, Rudolph. *Diet and Nutrition*. Himalyan Pres, Honesdale, Pensylvania. 1978.

Diamond, Harvey and Diamond, Marilyn. *Fit for Life*. Bantam Books, London. 1987.

PART THREE
THE PROFESSIONAL REFLEXOLOGIST

Practising reflexology at a professional level involves more than the giving of a treatment – although this is its heart and soul. In order to be in a position to give, the reflexologist must see to many other aspects. These include obtaining and maintaining safe, appropriate and legal business premises (if self-employed), furnishing the therapy room appropriately, attending to day-to-day administrative details, maintaining accurate accounts, and promoting her practice to the public. In addition and of great importance, today's reflexologist has a responsibility to hone and develop her skills, to constantly improve her knowledge of the subject and to continue developing herself as a professional and as a person. As reflexology gains a wider appeal, as more reflexologists are training to high professional standards, the profession is growing as a major force in the field of complementary medicine and is becoming more accepted within mainstream health care. Together, we professional reflexologists are committed to even higher standards of training, and reflexologists from all over the world are joining together to share experience and expertise for the greater benefit of their clients.

After working through this chapter you will be able to:

- understand the importance of drafting a business plan and where to get help
- understand your responsibilities for maintaining accounts, filing tax returns and paying National Insurance contributions
- know how to contact advisory services or helplines that can be of help to you in managing the business side of your reflexology practice
- begin to formulate ways of promoting your practice in the local community
- understand the value of giving talks to the public on reflexology and the important elements involved in public speaking.

Gaining a qualification in professional reflexology is a necessary first step to a successful practice. But it is only the first step. Working with clients is our goal and to achieve this takes a lot of hard work.

As complementary medicine is accepted more and more by the public, opportunities for giving reflexology increase. At the same time, there is increased competition as more practitioners are trained.

Identify your preferred place and style of practice

Perhaps the first thing you need to do is to decide what kind of reflexology you want to practise. For example, would you like to work independently in your own private clinic, with other complementary practitioners in a group practice, within a general practice surgery (this is increasingly a possibility), in a hospital, hospice, nursing home or in a recreation, health or holiday centre? Would you like to be on a self-employed or on an employee basis? It is possible in some areas to combine one or two of these. You may decide that you prefer to give some, or even all, of your treatments voluntarily; some reflexologists are in a position to donate their skills, for example to a local hospice. Many reflexologists like working from home, while others have a practice based on home visits to clients.

Bear in mind that there are differences between being self-employed and employed. If you are employed, your employer is responsible for National Insurance contributions, and for working out your tax as part of Pay As You Earn (PAYE). Safety and health regulations are also the employer's responsibility. However, while your money is not put at risk and you are not directly responsible for profits or losses, you may have little or no say in the running of the business. If you are self-employed, you are responsible for taxes, contributions, health and safety, as well as capital risks, but you can also enjoy creating your own enterprise.

If you are self-employed you also need to decide if you want to work full-time or only part-time. This will determine to what extent you promote yourself.

> **ACTIVITY**
>
> Start a file or folder to store all your business information in an orderly fashion.

If you decide to work from home, bear in mind that a room used exclusively for business may become liable for a business rate of tax, and liable for capital gains tax when the property is sold. On the other hand, you can claim the full cost of expenses associated with the room on your tax return.

> **ACTIVITY**
>
> With fellow students discuss and draw up a list of the advantages and disadvantages of :
>
> a) running a clinic from home b) working from a group practice of complementary therapists c) making home visits to clients.

Drafting a business plan

Before setting yourself up in business it is a good idea to create a business plan. Even if you don't need to show it to a bank manager, this encourages you to think realistically about what you need and do not need for your practice. Any bank will be able to advise you on drawing up a business plan. They usually require this as part of the application for a loan.

> **ACTIVITY**
>
> The Department of Trade and Industry produces booklets which can help small businesses. Call 0870 150 2500 and ask for copies of these relevant to your profession.

The information asked for on a business plan includes such things as: your training, qualifications and experience, a customer profile or idea of your target market, proposed charges or a comparison with competitor's charges, setting-up and running costs, projections about profits and income from the business, cashflow statements and forecasts. A cashflow forecast is a way of working out how much cash a business is likely to generate in a future period. After you have been in business, it can be calculated on the basis of past receipts and payments made on a regular basis. The cash flow itself is found in the difference between outgoings and receipts over a given period.

_____
_____
_____
_____
_____

BUSINESS DETAILS

Name of business
_____

Status of business

Type of business

Telephone

Date business began if you have already started trading

Business activities
_____
_____

PERSONAL DETAILS

Name

Address
_____

Telephone (home)	Telephone (work)
Qualifications	
	Date of birth

Relevant work experience
_____
_____

Business experience
_____
_____
_____

Details of personnel (if any)

Name	Name
Position	Position
Address	Address
Date of birth	Date of birth
Qualifications	Qualifications
Relevant work experience	Relevant work experience
Present income	Present income

What skills will you need to buy in during the first two years?
_____
_____

PERSONNEL

Estimate the cost of employing any people or buying any services you may need in the first two years

Number of people	Job function	Monthly cost	Annual cost

(Remember to include your own salary and those of any partners you may have in this calculation)

PRODUCT/SERVICE

Description of type of service to be offered
_____
_____
_____
_____
_____

continued

Contribution of individual services to total turnover

Service

_____

_____

_____

_____

_____ | Percentage contribution

(the figures in this column should add up to 100)

Break down the cost of equipment

EQUIPMENT | Cost

_____

_____

_____

_____

MATERIALS | Cost

_____

_____

_____

_____

_____

_____

_____

_____

_____

Where did you get your estimate from?

Material | Source

_____

_____

_____

MARKET

Describe your market

_____

_____

_____

Where is your market?

_____

Who are your customers?

_____

Is your market growing, static or in decline?

_____

Itemise the competitive products or services

Competitor's name

Competitor's product/service   1

Name _____ | Price

Strengths | Weakness

_____

_____

Competitor's name

Competitor's product/service   2

Name _____ | Price

Strengths | Weakness

_____

_____

Competitor's name

Competitor's product/service   3

Name _____ | Price

Strengths | Weakness

_____

_____

What is special about your product or service?

_____

_____

_____

Advantages of your product or service over competitor   1

_____

_____

continued

Competitor   2

Competitor   3

What is your sales forecast for the
*1st three months?

Treatments/products   Total value

*2nd three months?

Treatments/products   Total value

*3rd three months?

Treatments/products   Total value

*4th three months?

Treatments/products   Total value

(*These are assumptions)

Explain how you have calculated these estimates

Give details of any firm orders you have already taken

MARKETING

What sort of marketing do your competitors do?

Competitor   1

Competitor   2

Competitor   3

What sort of marketing or advertising do you intend to do?

Method   Cost

Why do you think that these methods are appropriate for your particular market?

Where did you get your estimates from?

Method   Source

PREMISES/EQUIPMENT/PRODUCT

PREMISES

Where do you intend to locate the business and why?

What sort and size of premises will you need?

What are the details of any lease, licence, rent, rates and when is the next rent review due?

What equipment and products do you require?

Is equipment bought or leased and how long is their life span?

On what terms will the products be purchased?

continued

RECORDS

Describe records to be kept and how they are to be kept up to date

OBJECTIVES

What are your personal objectives in running the business?

Short-term

Medium-term

Long-term

How do you intend to achieve them?

What objectives do you have for the business itself?

Short-term

Medium-term

Long-term

How do you intend to achieve them?

FINANCE

Give details of your known orders and sales (if any)

	Date	Orders sales	Details	Delivery date
1				
2				
3				
4				

Give details of your current business assets (if any)

Item	Value	Life expenctancy

What will you need to buy to start up and then throughout your first year?

Start up

Item	Value

Year 1

Item	Value

How will you pay for these?   Value   Date

Grants

Own resources

Loans

Creditors

continued

What credit is available from your suppliers?		
Supplier		

What are your loan or overdraft requirements?

What are you pulling yourself?

What security will you be able to put up?

OTHER
Accountant
Address
Telephone
Solicitor
Address
Telephone
VAT registration
Insurance arrangements

Adapted from: Good Practice in Salon Management by Dawn Mernagh-Ward and Jennifer Cartwright, Nelson Thornes Ltd.

Business help and advice

Many other agencies, besides banks, exist to help new businesses. Among the places offering free help are: the Training and Enterprise Council, Chamber of Commerce, Local Enterprise Agency, business enterprise trusts and small business advisory centres.

Business Link is a network of offices which provide a single point of access for all key local business support agencies, including the Training and Enterprise Council, Local Enterprise Agency, Chamber of Commerce and Local Authority. The address of local Business Link offices is in the telephone directory.

ACTIVITY

1 Write to three banks and ask them for some information on preparing a business plan. Compare the information from the banks with the sample provided here and draw up a plan which seems best suited to your practice.

2 Find out exactly which business start-up support agencies are active in your area. Contact each one and discover what help they can give you. Keep the information in your business file or folder.

1 What is Business Link?
2 How would you formulate a cashflow forecast once you have been in business for one year?
3 What are the differences between self-employment and employee status?

Planning

When you are planning the start of your practice, remember that in a business sense, practising reflexology involves more than just giving the treatment. In order to give the treatment you need to have secured such things as the worksite, transportation to work, possibly the equipment and overheads involved in running a clinic, even if yours is only a proportional contribution. In addition, keeping client records, ordering supplies and paying bills and promoting your business through talks and advertisements takes a certain amount of administration time which must be allowed for in your overall concept.

GOOD PRACTICE

From the beginning, set up a regular routine for your business administration. Do your paperwork, whether client records or your accounts, on a regular basis.

As people who just want to give a caring treatment it is easy to resent such considerations as not part of reflexology, but this is not a positive approach. We must remember that we do these things in order to enable us to give the treatments, not as an end in themselves.

Starting up

Once in business, you must notify:

1 Your local tax office.
2 Your local Social Security office.
3 Customs and Excise, if your annual turnover is above a certain amount.
4 Your local Job Centre, if you are registered with one.

Maintaining accounts
If you are self-employed you need to keep full and accurate records of all your business transactions. These include:

- all income received
- all business expenses incurred
- drawings for yourself
- any loans put into the business
- capital expenditure items.

This information is filed as an annual return with the Inland Revenue every year. These may be examined at any time so must be carefully and accurately kept. Bear in mind that accounts may also be required for reasons unconnected with tax, for example by your bank when considering an application for a business loan.

Income tax

Each year in April you will receive a Tax Return to fill in giving information on the year's earnings, any capital gains and your net profit – the amount left over after expenses and eligible deductions for the year. If your earnings exceed your tax allowances, the money you are allowed to earn each year before paying tax, you will be assessed and required to pay tax. Your allowance is calculated by the Inland Revenue on the basis of the information you supply them about your individual circumstances. The Inland Revenue will issue you with a Notice of Coding, or tax code which gives the amount of money you can earn tax free and detailing what benefits have been deducted.

It's a good idea to set money aside regularly to cover your yearly tax bill. Information about tax assessments and filing returns can be obtained from your local office of the Inland Revenue, and many local accountants offer free advice on the basics.

ACTIVITY

There is a helpline for those with problems relating to self-assessment: 0845 915 4515. Phone and ask if they will send you any information leaflets relating to self-employment. Keep these for reference.

National Insurance

Most people who work are liable to pay National Insurance contributions, unless they qualify for an exemption. Self-employed people are liable for two classes of contributions, Class 2 (paid towards benefits, except unemployment) and Class 4 (paid on profits and gains). Unless you have either been excused payment because of low earnings or are a married woman or a widow with reduced liability you must pay Class 2. These can be paid either quarterly every 13 weeks, or by direct debit every month.

Employers are responsible for Class 1, earnings-related contributions to the PAYE scheme. An employee can claim for sickness, invalidity, maternity, unemployment, and widow's benefit where appropriate, once enough contributions have accumulated.

ACTIVITY

Check with your Tax Office or a local accountant for more information about National Insurance. Ask about small earnings exceptions, and making and deferring payments.

VAT

Value Added Tax (VAT) is a government tax charged on most goods and services. Currently the rate is 17.5% for businesses with a taxable annual turnover of £54,000 or more. As giving reflexology is a service, it may be liable for VAT once the turnover from the business reaches the annual amount and the business must be registered for VAT with the local office. A registration number will be issued and true and accurate records must be kept on all business transactions. Every three months it will be necessary to fill in a VAT return form and where output tax exceeds input tax the difference will need to be paid to Customs and Excise.

ACTIVITY

1 Write to the Inland Revenue, Customs and Excise office and Social Security and ask for information leaflets relevant to being in business. Study the information and discuss it with your fellow students.

2 Call or write to a local accountant and ask if you can have a courtesy consultation. They are usually happy to provide free basic information. Find out whether it would be to your advantage or not to have your accounts handled by a professional.

Progress Check

1 What is VAT?
2 Why is it useful to formulate a business plan?
3 What is a notice of coding?
4 What is self-assessment?

Advertising and promoting your practice

Planning is essential when deciding ways to advertise and promote your practice. Give some thought to what type of clients you wish to attract, then you can make decisions about such things as: the appropriate medium for advertisements, as well as the style, tone and presentation so that you engage the audience's attention. Consider what are the five or six most vital pieces of information that should appear in any form of advertising for reflexology. Promotion needs to be cost effective as well and there are usually local avenues of free advertising. There are many ways to promote yourself besides advertising. A few of these are included here.

> **REMEMBER**
> Advertising should be in keeping with the code of practice and ethics of your professional association.

Suggestions for ways to promote your practice

- Offer to give one treatment free for every five treatments received.
- Offer treatments as birthday or Christmas presents, with an attractive card the giver can use which announces the gift treatment and gives details about yourself and how to book.
- Write letters introducing yourself to local groups such as the Women's Institute, National Women's Register, Weight Watchers, and support groups for such conditions as arthritis, and ME

(myalgic encephalomyelitis). Offer to give talks and demonstrations.

◆ Participate in any local complementary medicine 'fairs', though you need to check these out first to see how suitable they are and how productive they might be. If there are no such events, think about organising one yourself or with other local holistic practitioners.

◆ Create a business card and letter-headed stationery.

◆ Create a leaflet for distribution to the public. Research the best sites where you might leave your leaflets for free distribution.

◆ Write to your local GP practice manager introducing yourself, explaining reflexology and offering to arrange a meeting to discuss with them how reflexology might be useful to their patients. Restrict yourself to one or two conditions which are common and which usually respond well to reflexology and offer to do a trial period giving treatments for these. Such treatments may save the practice money on their prescription bills.

◆ Have a special day or half day a week in which you treat children and/or new mothers free. Have a special day for clients with a specific condition, such as asthma or pre-menstrual syndrome.

◆ When you open your practice, and whenever you have something substantially new of interest to the public, send a press release to the local papers to try and get them to cover the event. The press release should be very brief but contain essential information: your name, address and telephone number, time, date, address of the event and a brief description of its nature in such a way as to engage the interest of the editor. Try to find an interesting and new angle to your story.

ACTIVITY

With a group of fellow students discuss the following topics:

1 What are the advantages and disadvantages, and relative effectiveness of these advertising methods or media?

newspapers and magazines	notice boards (post office,
local radio	leisure centres, etc.)
direct mail	word of mouth
	letters to health clubs or
	companies

2 What types of publications would be particularly suitable for advertising reflexology?

3 What are the most vital points about reflexology or you the practitioner that need to be included in an advertisement?

4 What are some local groups and organisations which could be helpful to contact as useful conveyors of information about you and reflexology?

Giving talks

Giving talks to local groups of interested people is a very good way of promoting your practice and increasing public awareness of reflexology and complementary medicine in general. There are many organisations and groups looking for speakers at their regular meetings, for example, the Women's Institute, the National Women's Register, support groups for various conditions such as multiple sclerosis, arthritis, tinnitus, and civic groups such as the Rotary Club. More doctors, nurses and midwives are becoming aware of the benefits of complementary medicine; they want to know more and might be interested to have you as a speaker to their local associations.

Plan ahead and organise

As in any other activity, planning ahead is important. Before you even begin to outline your ideas, think about the kind of audience you have so you can direct the tone and level of the talk to them, to their interests and experience as far as you can. Being able to tie the information in the talk to specific aspects of their lives gives it more value.

Think about any posters or other visual material you could bring that will help you illustrate your ideas. As well as simply talking about reflexology, consider what activities you might also include, such as a demonstration of the technique, how this would be organised, and whether you think it's appropriate to get members of the audience to practise a technique on each other.

When planning your talk, put yourself in the position of members of the audience and think up questions they might have about reflexology then gear your talk to try to answer these question. For example, if there are doctors in the audience, they might be very concerned to know about levels of training and professionalism as well as about reflexology itself. Remember that many may be potential clients so they will want to know about costs, confidentiality, what is actually involved and often simply whether treatment is painful. Be prepared to answer such questions.

Write down all the ideas that you want to cover, then think through them again. Aim to have an introduction and a conclusion to round off the talk, and decide in what order you want to discuss your ideas. Use headlines to highlight the main points, and make some notes of the information in this order. It is perfectly acceptable to use notes when speaking. Before you give your first public talk, practise it on a helpful friend or family member or at least in front of a mirror. This will take out some of the anxiety about public speaking.

Insecurities

Giving talks to the public is daunting for many people, especially at first. It helps if you can start with small, familiar groups. The more talks you give, the easier it becomes. But there is always likely to be the odd question that comes as a surprise. The best approach is to speak from your own experience, including your life experience in general, give concrete, specific examples whenever possible, and above all don't be worried about admitting when something is outside your experience. It is perfectly acceptable to admit this, though it is helpful if you can think of someone to refer the questioner to for the answer.

> **REMEMBER**
> When speaking in public you are representing not only yourself but reflexology as a whole. A positive appearance and manner helps promote confidence and reflects well on the profession.

ACTIVITY

1 Brainstorm a list of questions you think an audience of midwives might ask about reflexology. What special areas would you need to concentrate on for this audience? Repeat this for a WI group. Compare your lists with those of two fellow students and make adjustments as needed.

2 With a partner, if possible, work out your answers for the following questions and then compare them:

   ◆ How would you answer the question 'How many treatments does a person usually need?'?

   ◆ Think of ten ways in which reflexology works that you might mention in a talk.

   ◆ How would you explain why some points on the feet feel tender?

   ◆ How would you answer the question 'How do I know if a practitioner is suitably qualified?'?

Key Terms

You need to know what these terms mean. Go back through the chapter or check in the glossary to find out.

◆ Business plan
◆ Tax return
◆ VAT
◆ Cashflow forecast
◆ Accounts

13 PROFESSIONAL DIMENSIONS

After working through this chapter you will be able to:

♦ understand the nature and scope of the legal responsibilities of a practitioner
♦ understand the need for insurance cover
♦ understand the need to conform to local requirements for businesses
♦ understand the advantages and privileges of belonging to a professional association
♦ know your responsibilities for reporting serious cases of disease or possibly dangerous symptoms
♦ appreciate the need for continuing professional development
♦ understand the need for maintaining high standards of ethics and conduct as a professional reflexologist.

Reflexology can be practised in a variety of settings, most frequently in a private clinic, the practitioner's home or a business address. Increasingly however, reflexology is being offered in residential, health, holiday or recreation centres. It is also becoming part of the health services and reflexologists can practise from GP surgeries and in hospitals. As reflexology takes a more established place in health care, professionalism and awareness of our legal responsibilities is very important.

Health and safety guidelines

Whatever the setting, a reflexology practice needs to conform to certain health and safety guidelines.

♦ Fire-fighting equipment is on site and kept in good working order. Equipment is readily accessible and suitable for fires that are likely to occur. Room contents do not obstruct exits.
♦ First aid equipment is on site and kept up to date. The reflexologist needs to have trained in first aid and to keep the certification up to date.
♦ The practice is accessible to disabled people.
♦ If practitioners are employed, the employer and employee must conform to the Health and Safety at Work Act 1974. The Act's main provisions are set out in the table below.

Insurance

Public Liability insurance and Professional Indemnity insurance is not statutory but is required of their members by responsible professional organisations because it provides important cover for reflexologists.

Employer	Safeguards as far as possible the health, safety and welfare of themselves, their employees, contractors' employees and members of the public.
	Ensures all equipment is kept up to standard.
	Ensures the environment is kept free of toxic fumes.
	Ensures safety equipment is regularly checked.
	Ensures all staff know safety procedures and provides safety information and training.
	Ensures safe systems of work.
Employee	Takes reasonable care to avoid injury to themselves and others.
	Co-operates with others.
	Does not interfere with or misuse anything provided to protect their health and safety.

Fig. 13.1 *The main provisions of the Health and Safety at Work Act 1974*

It covers the reflexologist for claims made by members of the public as a result of injury or damage to people or personal property resulting directly from the site of treatment or the treatment itself (this is termed 'professional negligence').

GOOD PRACTICE

Ensure that your practice is fully covered against Public Liability and malpractice – and keep the cover up to date.

Legal responsibilities

Local authority licence

When setting up a business giving reflexology treatments, application must be made to the Environmental Services department of your local authority for a licence to operate or a special treatment licence. Some, though not all, local authorities do require a licence for reflexology practices. The by-laws of your authority must be learned and observed. Licences are usually for a year, are charged for and allow an inspection by Environmental Services officers who have authority to fine or cancel registration of the business if it does not conform to the standards laid down by the authority. The aim is to protect the public by requiring practitioners to conform to the regulations as set forth in the licence.

REMEMBER
Keep first aid training up to date. Contact your professional organisation or local St John Ambulance Association for information about courses.

The Trade Descriptions Act 1968

Reflexologists are also bound by the provisions of the Trade Descriptions Act 1968. An important provision of the Act is the one against making any false statements as to services offered, or claims about the effectiveness of a treatment, and claims to cure or diagnose specific ailments.

In addition, Trade Descriptions Act laws list Prohibited Functions within the field of medicine which unqualified persons are forbidden to perform. These include: the treatment of venereal disease, and dentistry, midwifery and veterinary surgery. It is also an offence under the law to publicise or advertise any article or description so as to lead to the use of the article to treat certain diseases. These include: Bright's disease, glaucoma, diabetes, cancer, cataract, epilepsy or fits, tuberculosis, locomotor ataxia, paralysis.

Data Protection Act 1984

If a practitioner uses a computer to store personal data about clients, they must register with the Data Protection Registrar or be liable to prosecution. The Act only applies to information relating to living persons stored on computer. Information and forms are available from post offices. Registration is for three years and involves a fee. Clients who feel they are affected by lost or incorrect information or wrongful disclosure without consent may make a claim to the Registrar and are entitled to see the data relating to them.

Performing rights

If recorded music or a radio is played in a place of business, a fee is payable. For information contact the Performing Rights Society, 29–33 Berners Street, London W1T 3AB (tel: 0207 5805544) and/or Phonographic Performance Ltd, Ganton House, 14–22 Ganton Street, London W1F 7QU (tel: 0207 4370311). If radio or television broadcasts are used, similarly, the premises must hold a licence.

Children under 16

When treating a child under 16, the practitioner must also be careful. It is an offence under the law for a parent or guardian to fail to provide adequate medical aid for a child, and by treating a child who is not also under medical care, the reflexologist may be said to be 'aiding and abetting' an offence.

ACTIVITY

Write to your local authority Environmental Services department enquiring about the conditions which must be fulfilled to practise reflexology in your area.

1   If you treat a child, it is sensible to compose a brief statement for a parent or guardian to sign. This would document the fact that the parent has been warned by you that according to the law they should consult a doctor about the health of the child. Why is this procedure sensible?

2   What are some of the provisions of the Trade Descriptions Act which relate to reflexologists?

3   Describe what is meant by professional negligence.

4   Other than the local council, where else might you be able to find out if a Local Authority had licence requirements or procedures?

Professional life

Professional organisations

It is highly recommended that reflexologists belong to a good professional organisation. Some addresses are listed in the Resources section. Your teacher should also be able to advise you. Membership has numerous advantages, which should at least include the following.

- A register of professionally qualified members whose names can be given to members of the public enquiring for a reflexologist in their area.
- Reflexology is promoted, with accurate information being given to the media and the medical profession to educate them to the value of reflexology.
- A periodical journal is circulated to members which communicates information about various aspects of reflexology and provides a forum for discussion of issues and subjects of professional interest or relevance to members.
- Ability to obtain insurance at competitive rates.
- Sale of books and other items of use to practitioners.
- Organising of regional support groups for members.
- Support for professional development through an ongoing educational programme of seminars and workshops organised by the body.
- Promotion and development of high educational and training standards for practitioners.
- Assessment and accreditation of training courses to high professional standards and providing a list of such courses for information to prospective students.
- Keeping members informed of developments in the field of reflexology, and complementary medicine in general, at both national and international levels as monitored by the organisation.
- Supporting, monitoring and engaging in research projects into the benefits of reflexology.
- Working with other organisations in the field of complementary medicine for the benefit of professionals and the public.

Professional discipline

A good professional organisation will have in place a clear statement of investigative and, if necessary, disciplinary procedures to be followed in the event of a complaint being received by someone against a member practitioner. The aim of such procedures is to ensure that high standards of practice and ethics are adhered to by members in order to protect the public, but also to provide means by which the member may be enabled to raise his or her standard of treatment.

GOOD PRACTICE

Be discreet in conversations and in any promotional talking that you do, and in any literature or advertisements that you produce.

Referrals to other professionals

A qualified reflexologist always works within the limits of her own training and expertise. When faced with a client whose needs are assessed as being outside the range of the practitioner's expertise, in the client's best interest the reflexologist has no hesitation in referring the client to another practitioner – whether this be a medical physician, a practitioner of another complementary discipline, counsellor or other professional. New clients should be asked if they have consulted a doctor about their symptoms and, if they have not, be advised to do so. This advice should be recorded in the case record.

In addition, the reflexologist is obliged to report certain types of disease conditions to a doctor or medical authority. These include:

- sexually transmitted diseases (STDs)
- any bleeding reported in the stools, urine, phlegm from coughing, or vomit; vomit with dried blood (like coffee grounds); non-menstrual bleeding, vaginal bleeding with pregnancy or after a missed period
- pain in the eye or temples of elderly or rheumatic people, with local tenderness – sign of a possible stroke
- stiff neck and/or high fever, photophobia – possible sign of meningitis
- any sudden difficulty breathing, whether breathing is cut-off, rapid or laboured – sign of possible heart condition or severe respiratory condition
- drowsiness or loss of consciousness, dizziness, vomiting following an injury.

Continuing professional development

As discussed at the beginning of this textbook, basic training in reflexology is only the beginning. A good reflexologist is under an obligation to continue to develop professional skills in all areas by engaging in further training on a regular basis, at least bi-annually. Training may be specifically in reflexology skills, business skills, or in any area which has a direct bearing on the understanding of health and disease. Professional reflexology involves lifelong learning.

Attendance at further training seminars and workshops has an added advantage for the reflexologist. It is an opportunity to share experiences with fellow practitioners and to glean new insight and information from others' experiences. Such events usually stimulate the practitioner to try new approaches and think in new ways to the benefit of the practitioner and client alike.

Developing reflexology skills and expertise also involves continuing self-education, developing further our knowledge of ourselves, and our self-awareness. We can never know all there is to know, but we can continually extend our range of understanding. This allows us to practise and give to our clients from a neutral and safe space of inner calm and compassion.

Code of ethics

A good professional organisation will require that members abide by a professional code of ethics (code of coduct or code of practice). This will include such subjects as, for example, confidentiality, working within the limits of training, not prescribing or diagnosing, the duty to report infectious diseases and to advise clients to seek medical help for symptoms, keeping records of advice given, prohibitions about claims seeking to attract business unfairly, and bringing discredit on reflexology.

> **REMEMBER**
> The reflexologist accepts the responsibility to refer a client to the GP or other suitable practitioner if circumstances indicate this is necessary.

ACTIVITY

1 Obtain a copy of the code of ethics of the professional organisation to which you hope to belong. After studying the code, discuss the provisions with a group of fellow students, airing any uncertainties about the principles and becoming clear about what is expected.

2 Research some of the newer developments in reflexology such as Advanced Reflexology Training (ART), Reflexology and Meridian Therapy, Universal Reflexology, Precision Reflexology, Vertical Reflexology, Cranial-Sacral Reflexology, and others (obtain addresses from your tutor or reflexology organisations). Send for information or interview someone who has trained in or experienced these methods. Report on your results.

Progress Check

1 What is the intention of a code of ethics?
2 How does adhering to a code of ethics help protect both the practitioner and the client?
3 What are four advantages of belonging to a professional association?
4 Why does a professional reflexologist need to be committed to continuing education and training in her profession?

Complementary and Alternative Medicine (CAM) 2000 and beyond

Within the last few years in the UK, complementary medicine therapies, especially reflexology, have become recognised as valid forms of treatment in many cases and are very popular with the public. The Prince of Wales, long a supporter of CAM, was instrumental in founding the Foundation for Integrative Medicine, whose title is meant to highlight the fact that complementary medicine can and should be integrated into our national health-care systems. In addition, the government has been facilitating the work of the various professional bodies towards consolidation, with a view to agreeing training standards and course curricula, and mechanisms of public accountability. The House of Lords established a select committee to investigate complementary therapies and its report has been published (web address in *Resources and further reading*, page 268). Most of its recommendations are already in hand among professional reflexologists who have been co-operating to establish common standards of training and competency via the Reflexology Forum and Healthwork UK.

Research in CAM

The House of Lords Select Committee strongly recommended that an understanding of basic scientific research methods and outcomes should be included in training and that more research should be done in CAM so the public can use it with knowledge and security.

Research has been done into reflexology, most notably by Danish reflexologists over many years. However, historically it has not been emphasised or generally facilitated within the profession. This is now changing. Professional bodies are putting into place protocols and guidance, and encouraging and supporting their members to engage in research. As part of the mainstream, the research's style of language and writing needs to follow modern research standards. Likewise diseases or conditions are identified from the conventional medical perspective, as well as a holistic one.

Basic stages in research involve such things as:

- ♦ conception and focusing of the hypothesis to be tested
- ♦ identifying and developing the appropriate methodology
- ♦ writing a grant proposal, applying for and obtaining funding from the appropriate external funding body
- ♦ conducting the research, evaluating the results, drawing conclusions
- ♦ writing up the results and submitting the research for peer review
- ♦ publishing the results so others can benefit.

Conducting research is a difficult but very rewarding task. Although it may seem contrary to some of the principles of holism, if carefully designed this need not be so. It can be a means of methodical self-evaluation of our skills and professionalism as well as a means of discovering new areas for reflexology development or areas needing improvement. It can identify particular conditions that benefit consistently from reflexology. For example, recently conducted trials have shown reflexology to be of excellent benefit in childbirth. A new trial is exploring its benefits for infertility. Research can validate (or invalidate) the efficacy of a particular technique or combination of techniques. It can explore new methods in a coherent, organised way. Research can highlight areas where its application could inform conventional medicine, for example by showing cost-effectiveness of reflexology treatment relative to conventional care. In summary, research can be of benefit to both therapists and the public.

ACTIVITY

1 Find out more about the Foundation for Integrative Medicine and its activities or the House of Lords Select Committee Report. Make a report to your fellow students.

2 In a group, discuss the ethics of scientific research relative to a holistic therapy.

3 Using the internet or by writing to professional associations, try to find some research into reflexology that has been published and accepted. Review and evaluate it and make a report to your fellow students.

4 Find out the difference between quantitative and qualitative research. How could you use each in a reflexology trial?

5 Brainstorm an idea for a research trial.

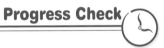

Progress Check

1 What are the benefits of conducting research?
2 Why is it important to use conventional language and style in formulating and writing up research?
3 Why might publishing one's research be important?

Reflexologists in Europe and worldwide

Through membership of a professional organisation the practitioner can be in contact with reflexologists from Europe and throughout the world. In 1994 the European Conference of Reflexologists was formed which organises and promotes biennial conferences of reflexologists from all over Europe where seminars are given, and workshops held. Different kinds of reflexology treatments are exchanged and communication and healing occur through the universal language of the feet.

This Conference is currently engaged in lobbying on behalf of reflexologists for legislation to be passed by the European Union to establish the principle of freedom of choice in health care. This in turn recognises the legitimacy of complementary/holistic medical disciplines and allows reflexologists to practise in every member state. Until such time as legislation is enacted, reflexologists need to be aware that a qualification from the UK does not automatically entitle you to practise or even to give treatments in a foreign country. If you wish to do so, you will need to learn about any local or national legislation covering such practice. You may obtain help from the country's professional reflexology association if there is one.

Reflexology is one of the disciplines most conducive to practice in a variety of settings and cultures. When we join together with reflexologists from other countries we exchange views and techniques, we share experiences and support each other. Finally we create a powerful force for positive change and the healing of our planet at all levels.

Key Terms

You need to know what these terms mean. Go back through the chapter or check in the glossary to find out.

- Referral
- Code of ethics
- Professional development
- Personal development

COMMUNICATION AND UNDERSTANDING YOUR CLIENT

After working through this chapter you will be able to:

♦ understand the term 'therapeutic space'
♦ practise creating therapeutic space whilst working with clients
♦ understand the importance of 'active listening'
♦ practise the component skills which make up active listening
♦ reflect on blocks to effective communication.

The way we work with clients reflects, in many ways, our own views and value system about other people and reflexology. If I am constantly telling people what is 'best' for them and what they 'should' do then I am essentially telling them that they are not capable of making their own choices and decisions.

Within any therapeutic relationship healing is not a passive process. It is not 'I', the reflexologist, who, through my skill and expertise, heals 'you' the client. Primarily, reflexology is about empowering clients to take charge of their own health; this requires an open, honest dialogue between reflexologist and client. Learning does not stop once you acquire the skills necessary to become a technically proficient practitioner. Reflexologists also need to possess a wider repertoire of human skills. It is to these skills that this chapter now turns.

> **REMEMBER**
> You need to link this chapter with the work you have done on the Consultation Process. Refer back to Chapter 3.

The human condition

'The reason why we have two ears and only one mouth is that we may listen the more and talk the less.'

Zeno of Citium

As individuals we all make assumptions about other human beings. However, when we work in a therapeutic setting, we need to be clear what these assumptions are for they will guide the way we work with our clients.

Basic assumptions about people help form the context for the reflexologist's relationship with the client.

Individuals need and deserve understanding and acceptance
Clients need to feel valued as people. This does not mean that you have to agree with their behaviour or condone what you may view as detrimental to their health. However, it is important 'to get into their shoes' and try and understand why a client continues to behave in a certain way. Human beings need acceptance and understanding before they can change.

> **REMEMBER**
> There is a Native American saying: 'Do not judge a person until you have walked in their moccasins for two moons'.

Human beings are capable of change
Clients have learned ways of being which do not always contribute to their optimum health. When individuals feel accepted they can

experiment with different options and ideas. Change is a slow process for many of us but it can occur when we feel supported and not judged, and when we set our own goals. For example, if both you and your client feel that it is important for their health to cut down on their coffee intake, make an agreement to do it gradually. Goals need to be realistic.

Human beings are experts on themselves

Each client who comes to us knows his or her own thoughts and feelings. They know their own anxieties and fears. They also know how to involve themselves in the healing process. We do not know 'better' than they do. However, they may need varying amounts of support to heal and that support may not just be from a reflexologist.

> **ACTIVITY**
> With another student discuss the three assumptions listed above. How do you feel about them? What are your assumptions about human nature? Jot them down and discuss them in a small group.

Listening

> *'It is as though she listened and such listening as hers enfolds us in a silence in which at last we begin to hear what we are meant to be.'*
>
> Lao-Tse

> **REMEMBER**
> When a client says to us 'Yes, that's it exactly' then we know that we have really heard them.

It is important to make the distinction between *hearing* and *listening*. Hearing is a physiological process involving sounds received by the ears and transmitted to the brain. Listening is a psychological process involving interpreting and making sense of another's meaning. When an individual feels that she has been 'really heard', it enhances the quality of communication and thus the whole relationship.

We are now going to look at and practise some of the skills which make up what is known as 'active listening'. However, a word of warning – they are not mechanical skills like riding a bike or driving a car. These skills will only be effective when taken in context with the following qualities:

- genuineness – being appropriately open about one's feelings, needs and ideas. Allowing the 'real self' to be seen
- non-possessive love – this involves respecting and supporting another person in a freeing way
- empathy – the ability to see and hear another person from their own perspective (walk in their moccasins!).

It is worth remembering that a person may have technically mastered the skills of communication but if they lack genuineness, love and empathy they will find their expertise underutilised.

For the purpose of this chapter active listening is broken down into three component parts – each part broken into specific skill areas. The component parts covered are:

- attending skills
- following skills
- reflecting skills.

Attending skills

These are *non-verbal* ways of showing your interest and involvement. It is these unspoken signals which will allow your client to feel safe with you and thus begin to express their needs.

Specific skills

Posture – we need to show physical openness and this may be done in a variety of ways. The reflexologist needs to face the client directly and sit in a relaxed (but not too relaxed!) way. Lean slightly forward to show interest and guard against crossing arms and legs to maintain this feeling of openness. Position yourself at what you feel is an appropriate distance. Remember not to crowd someone or move into their space too quickly. Chairs also need to be at the same height.

Eye contact – good eye contact shows interest and that you are trying to understand your client. Good listening involves 'softly focusing' on the client as opposed to staring at them. Clients may avert their gaze or look around the room when talking about a sensitive issue, but when they return to look at the reflexologist your eyes need to be still softly focused on them.

Non-distracting environment – you cannot give someone your undivided attention if there are constant distractions. Invest in a 'Do Not Disturb' sign for your treatment room and make sure your telephone is either unplugged or the answering machine is on.

Facial expression – initially your facial expression needs to be warm and welcoming. However, as your listening deepens, your expression needs to show that you have an understanding of what is being said, and needs to adjust itself accordingly. A good listener 'mirrors' the joy or sadness of the client with their own facial expression.

GOOD PRACTICE

Attending skills are non-verbal and show that we are listening with our whole being. Remember your posture, eye contact, facial expression and remember to provide a non-distracting environment.

Following skills

Following skills enable the listener to stay out of the way in order to let the speaker explain things from his or her own point of view. In other words, these are skills which help the *speaker* set the agenda NOT the listener.

Specific skills

Door openers are brief statements which show the speaker that you are available to listen. How many times have we gone into work or met a friend and known intuitively that all is not well? Individuals send very powerful non-verbal messages to indicate this – their body posture may show that they are burdened and you may get an overwhelming sense of anxiety. A door opener allows them the opportunity to talk.

Typically 'door openers' have four parts:

1   A description of the other person's body language, for example 'I can't help but notice that you seem a little anxious today'.
2   An invitation to talk, for example 'I'm not doing anything this lunch time. I'm around if you'd like to talk'.
3   Silence – to allow them to think about this and take up the opportunity if they choose to.
4   Attending skills – eye contact, facial expression, and a posture of involvement. All the non-verbal signals which show that you are concerned about them.

Encouraging statements are brief verbal expressions designed to encourage the client to start talking. They need to be kept to the minimum to allow the speaker to explore the area they wish to talk about. They help the speaker continue speaking. Whilst the listener may not say much, these minimal encouraging statements show the speaker that their world view is being validated. The most obvious one is the 'mm -hmm', but others are 'I see, go on, then . . ., tell me more . . ., really . . ., ah . . ., oh . . ., and . . . ?' These encouraging statements are neutral and imply neither agreement nor disagreement, rather they allow the speaker to explore the subject that they are talking about whilst being actively listened to.

Questions There are two important things to remember about questions within the context of active listening. They need to be infrequent and it is advisable to keep them as open as possible. Too many questions may lead the speaker to feel that she is under interrogation and open-ended questions allow for further exploration of the topic, for example, 'How do you feel about that?', 'What do you think that was about?'.

> **REMEMBER**
> Following skills include door openers, encouraging statements and questions.

Reflecting skills

Here the listener restates either the emotion and/or the essence of what the speaker has said. This shows an *active understanding* of the world of the speaker.

Specific skills

Paraphrasing is useful because if done effectively it cuts through the clutter of what has been said and really gets to the heart of the issue.

Client: I just don't know what's wrong. I've been crying all day.

Reflexologist: You're feeling low and can't seem to pinpoint why.

A good paraphrase often starts with the pronoun 'you' showing an understanding of the speaker's worldview.

Reflecting feelings is a skill which involves mirroring the emotional content back to the speaker. A good way is to pick up their feeling words and phrases.

Client: I just knew that my blood pressure had dropped. I wasn't at all worried about having it taken this time.

Reflexologist: It sounds like you're confident that things have stabilised.

It has been said that when we reflect feeling effectively 'we are responding to the speaker's music and not just to their words'. This allows the speaker to listen inwardly to their own emotions. Remember many people say one thing verbally but their bodies are saying something quite different – reflecting feelings allows you to check this out with the speaker.

Summaries may be viewed as longer paraphrases. They are particularly useful for the reflexologist to bring together the key points of the initial consultation. It gives an overview of the presenting issues and a clue to where your work together may start, for example:

Reflexologist: From what you have said the key areas which you seem to want to work on are . . .

They may also help during the treatment programme, allowing you to refocus or prioritise different issues, for example:

Reflexologist: I have been thinking about the last treatment and was wondering if you would like to continue working on . . . or would you like to perhaps concentrate on another area?

> **REMEMBER**
> Reflective skills are skills which allow the client to see that you have a real grasp of their situation. You offer back to the speaker what they have said – this enables you to check that you have really understood in a gentle way. The three skills discussed here are paraphrasing, reflecting feelings and summarising.

> **GOOD PRACTICE**
> You are a reflexologist not a counsellor. Don't get out of your depth. Any deep emotional problems need to be referred to a counsellor. Make contact with one locally so you can refer with confidence.

Blocks to communication

There are several pitfalls that the reflexologist should avoid.

Diagnosing – don't play the emotional detective or the amateur psychologist. Diagnosis is a form of labelling and not helpful.

Advising – this implies you know best.

Reassuring – you may feel that it is important to make a person feel better by reassuring them. However, what it may do is block a communication of true feelings. To say 'You'll be OK' or 'You'll feel better after this treatment' may not allow the client to express what they need to say.

Finally, remember: 'The gentle and sensitive listener is adept at the art of creating safety and a space for sharing that allows others to express their needs. This kind of listener observes the subtle language of the heart within others, respecting the appropriate timing needed for the trust to be present between the speaker and the listener. Hearing with the eye, nose, ears and heart of the spirit is how the astute listener reaches out to others, allowing healing to occur.' (Jamie Sams, *Earth Medicine – Ancestors' Ways of Harmony for Many Moons*).

ACTIVITY
Listening in threes

1 In threes, discuss the skills which make up active listening. (allow about 5 minutes).

2 Decide who is going to be the listener, the speaker, the observer. Ask the speaker to talk for 5 minutes on a joyful occasion. The listener needs to use the appropriate listening skills. The observer needs to jot down which skills were used competently and which ones need working on. Share the feedback and experience as a threesome. Swap roles to enable each person to experience each role.

 Progress Check

1 Explain the difference between hearing and listening.
2 What are attending skills?
3 What are following skills?
4 What are reflecting skills?

Key Terms

You need to know what these terms mean. Go back through the chapter or check in the glossary to find out.

- Door openers
- Encouraging statements
- Paraphrasing
- Summarising
- Blocks to communication

APPENDIX 1

Common conditions and reflexology

This appendix is provided for reference. It aims to describe some of the conditions that clients may present with – as they are medically understood. With this knowledge, the reflexologist can better appreciate what clients tell them about their symptoms and understand any medical treatments the client may be having, for example, why a client is on a particular medication. The reference is in no way intended to be exhaustive nor to be used to diagnose conditions, which would be contrary to professional ethics and to the whole viewpoint of this book. Serious medical conditions should always be referred to a medical practitioner for care.

In addition to describing the condition, suggestions are made as to which reflexes could be worked which might aid recovery. These are not intended as recommendations to give treatment, nor to be prescriptive nor to cover all the possible reflexes that might be involved. They are offered to give the reflexology student something to consider when beginning to decide what to treat. The nature and condition of the individual client are always taken into account and the reflexologist treats according to her assessment of the individual's needs, and in consultation with the client and a physician where necessary.

Holistic interdependency: the body as synergy

Although a symptom or condition may be primarily located in a particular part of the body, it is not isolated. Holistically, its imbalance will be interrelated and linked with the functions and health of other organs and systems. In this section, after describing a condition, suggestions are made of other reflexes which could be worked to aid the recovery. These are not intended to be prescriptive or to cover all the possible related reflexes, but to encourage the student to think holistically when treating, mindful of the interdependency of the body's many aspects. The client's individual nature and imbalance are also important considerations and the reflexologist treats according to each person's needs and, when necessary, in consultation with the physician.

For good information on disease conditions, consult:

Balch, James F. and Balch, Phyllis A. *Prescription for Nutritional Healing*. Avery Publishing, New York. 1999.
Ball, John. *Understanding Disease*. C.W. Daniel, Saffron Walden. 1990.
Murray, Michael and Pizorno, Joseph. *Encyclopedia of Natural Medicine*. Little Brown & Company, New York and London. 1990.

Conditions involving imbalance of the nervous system

The nervous system works in conjunction with the endocrine system to maintain the body's homeostatic balance and to respond to and – just as important – recover from stress. For this reason we suggest always working the endocrine reflexes in conditions of the nervous system. See page 131. Reflexes for the nervous system, especially all the spinal nerves, and specifically those related to the area concerned, should be worked as back-up for any condition, because increasing positive nerve energy to the muscle, joint, or organ plays an important part in recovery. Thus we use a holistic approach in treatment.

Conditions of the sensory organs: eyes, ears, nose

The reflexes for the sense organs, and the nerves feeding them, i.e. the cranial nerves, may also be worked as required in certain conditions, for example, eye problems, ear problems, smell or nasal problems, taste problems. Work the head area reflexes to access these nerves as well as the specific reflex points for ears, face, eyes, nose. Work any related areas.

Ear and throat conditions
Reflexes: the ears and nerves supplying them; additionally the throat/neck for the Eustachian tubes, all the toes, the lymphatics, the respiratory system if involved; the kidneys. If ears or throat are inflamed, work the adrenals and diaphragm. **Back-up reflexes:** the eliminative channels.

Middle ear infections
Germs from the Eustachian tubes infect the middle ear, pus builds up causing inflammation and pain, either acute or chronic. The concern is if it bursts the eardrum or spreads to the mastoid process. Holistically speaking, it is seen as a result of excess mucus in the area which becomes the focus for infection. Cleansing measures are used, especially a cleansing diet free of mucus-forming foods (for example, dairy products and junk food).

Reflexes include: ear, nose throat/neck, Eustachian tubes, lymphatic system (breast and neck area), lungs, endocrine system (adrenals for infections, pituitary for stimulating release of endorphins), cranial nerves. **Back-up reflexes**: all eliminative channels.

Outer ear infection
Infection, with pain, tenderness, redness, involving the outer ear canal, possibly with an abscess. May be brought on by swimming (excess damp).

Reflexes: same as for middle ear infection.

Glue ear
Eustachian tubes become blocked and allow accumulation of sticky fluid behind eardrum and loss of hearing. Repeated antibiotics for ear infections can contribute to this condition.

Reflexes: same as for middle ear infections.

Tinnitus
Ringing and other noises in the ears. May be associated with Ménière's disease also (fluid build-up in inner ear, causing pressure leading to dizziness, loss of balance, muffled hearing). Traditional medicine links this with a weakness of kidney/adrenal energy.

Reflexes: ears, neck, throat/Eustachian tubes, lymphatics, kidney and adrenals. **Back-up reflexes**: the eliminative channels.

Nose conditions

Reflexes: nose area (front of big toe), nerves to the nose; respiratory area if involved, lymphatics and eliminative channels. *See also* Respiratory system (page 134).

Headaches

Headaches can come from many factors, nervous tension could be one of them. Consider that headaches can be caused by imbalances in one or or more of the following and work appropriate reflexes accordingly:

- poor digestion/constipation
- poor or congested lymph circulation
- menstrual imbalance in women
- liver congestion, especially for migraine
- eye strain, for migraine
- neck, jaw or spinal (mid-back, shoulder) tension.

Consider what factors in the person, or the person's life may be contributing to the creation of headaches. Do they tend to strive after perfection or are they workaholics? Often migraines come when a very active person suddenly gets the chance to relax. Are they depressed and tense? Are they repressing anger? Cause could be dietary; some people are allergic to some foods (for example, chocolate, fatty, fried foods) which trigger the headache or migraine. Consider advising a cleansing diet. With migraine, sometimes eating as soon as the migraine is felt starting up, reduces its length and severity.

Sinus congestion headaches are often caused by excess mucus and poor digestion. Work the lymphatic reflexes and sinus points plus face, ears and neck, and suggest a cleansing diet.

Toxins in the colon can cause an occipital headache. Work the stomach and intestines and colon reflexes and recommend a cleansing diet.

Environmental causes also include factors at work or home which may lead to chronic muscle strain or tension. Ask about such things as how they sit at a desk, and what repetitive jobs they have to do. Changing the situation can remove the cause of the headaches.

Reflexes: the head area itself, site of the painful symptom.
Back-up reflexes: neck/occiput area, shoulder area, base of spine, whole spine, diaphragm/solar plexus, pituitary, thyroid and adrenal glands.

Include such reflexes as large and small intestine, sigmoid, liver-gall bladder, lymph.

Auxiliary treatment: self-reflexology, dietary changes, yoga, relaxation exercises. Bach flower remedies; taking time out for oneself; breathing exercises, including observing if one nostril has a more forceful discharge than the other. If so, close that nostril and breathe through the other until the headache subsides.

Insomnia
Disturbed sleep or inability to get to sleep.

Contributing factors include the diet, for example, too much tea or coffee; drinking liquids too late at night (especially the elderly, or pregnant women); digestive imbalances; emotional disturbance (worries, fears, or expectations which create an overactive mental state; depression, loneliness); too much activity late at night (reading and watching TV are very stimulating to the nervous system).

Reflexes: diaphragm/solar plexus, adrenal glands, spine. (Balancing occiput and sacrum.) **Back-up reflexes**: consider that poor sleep can be due to multiple factors. Question and observe your client and think out what are the causes for that individual and treat accordingly.

Auxiliary treatment: dietary changes, breathing and relaxation exercises. Bach flower remedies. Self-reflexology.

Tension, low vitality, fatigue
Residual tension in the muscles can lead to pain and fatigue.

Reflexes: same as for the nervous system, site of the particular tension, for example neck; plus all glands, especially adrenals but including reproductive; immune system (see Chapter 8). Circulatory system (heart-liver and lungs), the hypothalamus, kidneys and eliminative channels.

Sciatica
This sensation of pain at any or all points along the sciatic nerve can be due to several factors. Work reflexes accordingly, always including the diaphragm for pain. Possible causes vary.

1   Postural, for example, twisted pelvis, long leg syndrome, traumas (pregnancy, birth). Examine the patient's posture.
     Reflexes: spine, especially neck and sacrum/L5, sciatic loop around middle of heel; pelvic and hip area for gluteal muscles which can be tense and pulling the pelvis out of line.
2   Congestion: it has been known for sciatica to be caused or influenced by constipation, which creates congestion and pressure on the nerve as it comes out of the sacrum-L5.
     Reflexes: large and small intestines, especially sigmoid colon/rectum/anus, liver-gall bladder, diaphragm and solar plexus.

Auxiliary treatment: pelvic and back exercises, yoga, massage, self-reflexology. Cleansing diet (see Chapter 11).

Nervous system pathologies
These include such conditions as Bell's palsy, facial neuralgia, multiple sclerosis, Alzheimer's disease, epilepsy. The specific spinal reflexes for nerves to the site of the symptoms, e.g. brain, cervicals, muscles, etc. would be worked, if these are known. In addition, work the brain/big toe area and the neck reflexes. **Back-up reflexes**: include stress reflexes, endocrine reflexes and five eliminative channels.

Bell's palsy
A temporary paralysis of the muscles on one side of the face caused by a swelling of the facial nerve as it exits from the cranium. Pain in the ear,

and inability to close the eye may also be present. Usually clears of its own accord within 2 weeks. Orthodox treatment is steroidal.

Reflexes: face, big toe, all toes. Whole spine, ears, eyes. Diaphragm and solar plexus, adrenals.

Multiple sclerosis

Damage to the insulating sheath (myelin) of the nerve fibres causing disruption to nerve impulses, and formation of scar tissue. Progression of the disease is usually slow but causing gradual loss of various muscles, often in a pattern of decline, then some remission, followed eventually by more decline. Muscles affected early include those of the eyes, limbs, and urinary system. Believed to be brought on by shock or trauma to an already weakened nervous system. Depression, anxiety and irritability are obviously associated with this condition.

Reflexes: spine for nerves, brain for central nervous system, adrenals and all glands. Reflex to the site of any spasms, pain, numbness, loss of function, for example kidney and bladder.

Auxiliary treatment: Bach flower remedies, gluten-free diet, cleansing diet, kitcheree (see Chapter 11).

Epilepsy

An electrical event in the brain in which recurrent excessive electrical discharges from some nerve cells overwhelm the functioning of neighbouring cells, causing in some cases, loss of consciousness, falling, spasms and stiffness. Mild forms are called 'petit mal', more severe, 'grand mal'; also distinguished as focal – affecting just one part of the body; or lobal – affecting one lobe of the brain and causing uncharacteristic behaviours. Orthodox treatment is anticonvulsant drugs.

Reflexes: brain, spinal nerves, diaphragm/solar plexus, neck/throat, thyroid and all glands. **Back-up reflexes**: ileo-caecal valve, intestines.

Conditions involving imbalance of the endocrine and immune systems

Hypoglycaemia or low blood sugar

Many people are affected by periods of low energy, feelings of dizziness, confusion, or palpitations and a possible cause of this is low blood sugar. The pancreas has lost some of its ability to respond adequately to the demands made by the tissues for sugars.

Reflexes: pancreas, liver, all glands, digestive organs. **Back-up reflexes**: eliminative channels, spinal nerves, diaphragm/solar plexus.

Auxiliary treatment: many sufferers benefit from a diet rich in complex carbohydrates and from eating small amounts of food at frequent intervals to keep the sugar level in the blood more constant. Cleansing and wholefood diets will also help, as will flower remedies.

Diabetes mellitus

There are two main types, juvenile onset and adult onset. In juvenile diabetes the pancreas fails to function at an early age, perhaps because of a genetic defect, or auto-immunity; it fails to grow properly so can't keep up with the growing demands of an active life. The person will be insulin dependent throughout life. Reflexology can play an important role in helping the body to maintain its highest level of functioning and inhibiting the deterioration process. It is possible that with reflexology insulin intake may be kept at a lower level.

In adult onset, there are also two types, non-insulin dependent and insulin dependent. In the first type the pancreas' ability to produce adequate insulin has become impaired, but the blood sugar levels can be regulated by very careful attention to exercise and diet in order to reduce weight (less tissue, less need for insulin to meet its demands) and oral anti-diabetic drugs. In the second type, the person must take insulin injections (self-administered) as well as carefully monitoring the diet and sugar intake. Reflexology can be a help in either of these conditions, again inhibiting progress towards more extensive pathology, and in helping maintain optimal functioning of the other systems of the body, such as the circulation, peripheral nerves and vision, which are also affected by diabetes.

Stress is a major contributor to diabetes; blood sugar imbalances are affected by stress. Reducing tension through reflexology helps normalise and restore homeostasis. Sensitivity and good counselling skills are needed with these patients. They can be easily discouraged or lose the motivation to stick to their diet. Encourage them on both these fronts and to commit to a regular schedule of reflexology treatments to maintain momentum and inhibit deterioration.

Reflexes: pancreas, liver, digestive organs, adrenals and all stress and immune reflexes. Spine for nerves to these areas.

Auxiliary treatment: flower remedies; cleansing and wholefood diet, relaxation and breathing techniques, stress management; regular exercise, both moderate aerobic and yoga, t'ai chi.

Hypo- and hyperthyroidism

Whichever the person suffers from, reflexology can help to normalise function. It can be a good back-up to orthodox treatment and may reduce the amount of prescribed drugs (Thyroxin).

Many people show a range of symptoms of low thyroid (hypo-thyroidism) including weight gain, fatigue, poor memory, mental apathy. While not clinically ill, they may be suffering from borderline or slightly low hypothyroid function. This is not recognised by many doctors, though some are willing to authorise the tests necessary to detect it. If, through working the reflexes, you suspect this may be the reason for the client's symptoms, you can suggest they request a test through their GP.

Signs of hyperactivity (Graves' disease) include: exhaustion, insomnia, weight loss even though appetite increases, palpitations, nervousness, dry skin. The thyroid controls the general metabolic rate of the body processes, so we can see why these symptoms arise. Always refer patients to their GP for checks if you suspect this situation; but encourage them to continue reflexology which can help normalise this gland.

Signs of hypo-activity include: low blood pressure and heart rate, low body temperature, fatigue, weight gain. More serious are goitre, cretinism and myxoedema (thickening of the skin). Hypothyroidism is often missed in diagnosis.

Reflexes: thyroid and helper area for thyroid, all glands, spinal nerves to these. **Back-up reflexes**: diaphragm.

Weight problems

The goal of treatment is to normalise weight for that individual's natural build, not to force the body to conform to social images. At the same time, being overweight can adversely affect other conditions. Being underweight can also affect health in numerous ways so it is important to normalise weight.

Reflexes: thyroid-parathyroids and entire endocrine system, liver and digestive organs, all eliminative channels, especially kidneys; the spine for nerves to all these organs. Diaphragm/solar plexus. **Back-up reflexes**: stress reflexes, especially adrenals.

Stress

Review the discussion on stress in the Introduction; note that poor eating habits and allergic reactions both contribute to and reflect stress.

Reflexes: any specific site of known stress, for example, shoulders/neck, back, stomach. Adrenals and all glands, diaphragm/solar plexus, liver, kidney, lymph and eliminative channels; spinal nerves to these organs.

Auxiliary treatment: breathing and relaxation exercises, general relaxation techniques. Cleansing diet to eliminate allergenic factors and allow the digestive system to rebalance. Bach flower remedies, self-reflexology. Self-examination – what factors in my life are increasing my stress? Conditions at work, for example, what changes can I make to reduce/resolve these? How do I create stress for myself unnecessarily? How do I contribute to my own stress by my lifestyle, diet, emotional state, thought patterns? Work out a programme with your clients for decreasing these factors in their lives.

Immune compromised diseases (HIV, AIDS)

See also Lymphatic conditions (page 229).

Reflexes: endocrine glands in all cases, specific areas as symptoms appear, lymphatic glands. **Back-up reflexes**: include eliminative channels, diaphragm/solar plexus, whole spine and liver.

Auxiliary treatment: see above for Stress.

ME or Myalgicencephalomyelitis or Post-Viral Fatigue syndrome, Epstein-Barr syndrome

Little recognised until recently, partly because symptoms can belong to any number of complaints, ME is believed to result from the presence of a virus in muscles, causing low grade, chronic infection. Symptoms follow a viral infection such as flu or glandular fever and include complete fatigue/lassitude, muscle and joint pains, tingling, numbness, cold extremities, pallor, inability to concentrate, depression, memory loss, anxiety, digestive problems, headaches, poor immunity and allergic reactions. Symptoms can come and go, vary considerably, and last about four years. The programme for treatment must be multi-faceted and include diet, cleansing, and building up of the immune system.

Reflexes: liver, digestive system, glands, stress reflexes, immune reflexes, symptom sites, spine/nerves, diaphragm.

Auxiliary treatment: cleansing diet, kitcheree, wholefood diet/alkaline diet/Hay diet (Chapter 11). Relaxation exercises, gentle exercise/yoga/t'ai chi. Referral to homeopath, herbalist, Ayurvedic practitioner, nutritionist. Manual lymph drainage massage.

Lowered immunity

See also Stress (above). **Reflexes**: endocrine glands, lymphatic reflexes and spleen in all cases of lowered immunity, either for no clear cause, or from such conditions as ME. **Back-up reflexes**: include liver and eliminative channels.

Auxiliary treatment: suggest reflexology to your clients after bouts of infections and influenza or colds, to help strengthen the immune system and eliminate the toxins which probably caused them in the first place. Cleansing diet, wholefood diet and supplements, self-reflexology, Bach flower remedies, rest and recuperation, gentle, non-competitive exercise yoga, t'ai chi, etc.

Adrenal hypo- and hyper-function

With repeated stimulation from stress, these glands at first become a bit hyperactive (alarm reaction); people can even become addicted to the sensation resulting from adrenalin flowing through the system. However, repeated alarm stage reactions with no allowance for discharge of the energy created weakens the body eventually. Coffee, especially, over-stimulates the adrenal glands. The adrenal reflexes can feel acutely tender under any stressful circumstances or in the presence of caffeine intake.

Prolonged stress can lead to adrenal exhaustion – the adrenals have become weakened through overuse. Here the person may feel tired and that 'batteries have run-down'. This is the common 'burn out' syndrome. Reflexes may feel either tender or not tender at all! It is important to work the adrenals and all glands, in both these conditions.

Reflexes: adrenals, and all glands, eliminative channels. Diaphragm/solar plexus, spinal nerves to these areas.

Auxiliary treatment: same as for Stress (page 223).

Conditions of imbalance in the respiratory system

Colds, coughs

Occasional colds and coughs are signs that the body is undergoing a cleansing process. Reflexology can be a great help in this situation, supporting the body's own purpose.

Reflexes: the eliminative channels, nervous system, diaphragm/solar plexus to enhance rest and relaxation. Advise on diet, rest.

Upper respiratory tract conditions: sinusitis, polyps, tonsillitis

These conditions reflect the fact that mucus, congestion and/or toxicity in the body have reached such a level that organs in the second line of defence become involved. The body creates the inflammation, with its accompanying pain and swelling, sometimes discharge, to deal with the imbalance.

Reflexes: eliminative channels, especially the lymphatics. Site of symptoms such as sinus, nose, throat. **Back-up reflexes:** adrenals.

Auxiliary treatment: advise rest and cleansing diet. Bach flower remedies, self-reflexology.

Acute lower respiratory tract infections
Bronchitis

Inflammation of the bronchi, causing wheezing with thick yellow sputum and possibly coughing blood.

Reflexes: respiratory system in general. Lymphatics, eliminative channels. **Back-up reflexes:** stress reflexes, including adrenal glands. Advise on diet, rest.

Influenza

A viral infection involving fever, muscle aches and pains, respiratory congestion with either dry or mucus cough. Can be dangerous in elderly people, those with a history of chronic lung disease or smokers, due to risk of secondary bacterial infection (pneumonia).

Reflexes: all respiratory, all eliminative channels, especially lymphs. **Back-up reflexes:** stress reflexes, adrenals and all glands.

Pneumonia

This takes various forms and is due to the presence of pneumococcal bacteria, and the body's attempts to deal with it by creating high fever with flushed, dry skin, chills, aching and malaise with coughing. Breathing may be shallow and painful if the pleura, the lubricating membrane surrounding the lungs, is involved. This condition can seriously debilitate people for weeks afterwards. It will be rare for a reflexologist to treat during the acute stage of pneumonia, but advise clients to come in for a series of treatments after the acute phase has been treated medically.

Reflexes: respiratory system, eliminative channels, immune and stress reflexes. Advise cleansing diet (Chapter 11), adequate rest and recuperation.

Pleurisy

An acute infection of the pleura. This causes extreme pain and possibly clear fluids pouring into the pleural space. The danger is that the fluids compress the lungs or change to pus. Pleurisy usually results from a previous infection such as TB or some other serious condition.

Reflexes: treat as above for pneumonia, after client has received medical treatment.

Chronic respiratory conditions
Chronic bronchitis

Repeated attacks of bronchitis are often triggered by allergies, air pollution, dust, cigarette smoke, social factors, reduced immunity. These so damage the cilla lining the bronchioles that they cease to evacuate the waste products and debris in the tract. This then builds up to cause a permanent irritation of the mucosa. The weakened, toxic tissue becomes more susceptible to infections and further deterioration, and oedema. The result is coughing, haemoptysis (spitting blood or bloody mucus), wheezing due to reduced air passages, swellings and loss of lung surface to receive and expel air. Eventually it is more difficult to exhale than inhale completely, carbon dioxide cannot escape and remains in the blood causing cyanosis (blue colouration) and sluggishness.

Reflexes: respiratory system, immune, stress, and eliminative channel reflexes, nerves, glands.

Emphysema

Causes are similar to chronic bronchitis, but in some individuals deterioration tends towards reduced alveoli, with resulting breathlessness, and compensation through rapid breathing or puffing, usually with over-inflated chest. Individuals tend to be extremely thin, and wasting.

Reflexes: respiratory system, immune, stress, and eliminative channel reflexes, nerves, glands.

Asthma

This is a very complex condition involving emotional and psychological as well as purely physical factors. The nervous system, endocrine glands – especially the adrenals – as well as the lungs and diaphragm are greatly involved. Emotions such as anxiety, fear and/or lack of feeling loved are likely to contribute. With the sense of lack of adequate breath, a vicious circle is initiated of fear/anxiety-tension-narrowing of the bronchioles. If excess mucus accumulates in the bronchi, this too narrows or blocks the passages, so diet and cleansing are important factors. Eventually the whole system is involved and weakened.

Asthma may be set off by an allergic reaction, or by drugs, exercise, emotional upsets, any sudden changes, even in weather – all can be stressors. Symptoms are wheezing, breathlessness, tight feeling in the chest. In some people there is an inherited tendency, appearing in childhood, to allergic reactions which release histamines which constrict and swell the airways. Then expiration tends to collapse the bronchioles further and trap air inside alveoli which also swell, producing the characteristic wheeze and difficulty exhaling during an acute attack. This type of asthma often subsides as children enter adolescence – the 'growing out of it' effect – probably due to endocrine activity at this time.

In other individuals, especially women, asthma appears later, though again can be prompted by allergies to food additives, aspirin or non-steroidal anti-inflammatory drugs, even exercise. General wheezing becomes established and attacks occur within this pattern.

Think about the subtle causes of this problem. Why is the person feeling insecure, afraid, either in specific relationships or in relation to the world in general (hypersensitivity to environment)? How healthy is their sense of self-esteem? What traumatic events could act as triggers – whether during birth, early infancy/childhood or later (for example divorce, bereavement)?

Reflexes: respiratory system, diaphragm/solar plexus, eliminative channels, stress and immune reflexes (especially thymus and adrenals), nerves, thoracic spine, glands. **Back-up reflexes**: ileo-caecal valve.

Auxiliary treatment: flower remedies, cleansing diet, relaxation techniques, breathing exercises, especially pranayama (yoga breathing exercises), regular exercise. Enhance self-confidence.

Hay fever, allergic rhinitis

An allergic reaction to airborne irritants in which the body produces histamines which draw fluid to the site of the attack in an effort to flood it away. This creates redness, swelling, repeated sneezing, itching or tingling in the eyes, nose and throat mostly. Treatment is not just to avoid the irritant – if possible – but to try to cleanse and balance the whole body, so the over-reaction won't occur.

Reflexes: eyes, nose, throat, respiratory tract, adrenals, ileo-caecal valve. **Back-up reflexes**: diaphragm/solar plexus, all eliminative channels, glands, stress reflexes.

Auxiliary treatment: cleansing diet, flower remedies.

Conditions involving imbalance of the lymphatic system

Skin conditions

See also Imbalance of the Skin (page 248).

These can come from a number of causes such as lowered functioning of the respiratory and kidney eliminative channels, liver congestion, endocrine imbalances (for example at puberty or with adrenal hyperactivity), or emotional issues; but the lymph too plays an important role, because it is responsible for keeping all cells cleansed and nourished, and so we have chosen to place these problems under this section.

Basically, most skin problems arise because toxins that should be eliminated via the five eliminative channels are not fully cleansed from tissues, therefore the body chooses to try and eliminate them via the skin. This is why it is important to activate the eliminative channels and the liver, which also neutralises toxins in the blood. This is true of both acne and eczema, as well as boils and cysts.

Reflexes: eliminative channels, stress, liver, endocrine system and the nervous system.

Auxiliary treatment: cleansing diet, exercise, sweating therapy if appropriate.

Tonsillitis, swollen adenoids, swollen lymph nodes of neck axilla or groin, glandular fever

Reflexes: lymph, eliminative channels, adrenal glands.
Back-up reflexes: immune and stress.

Oedema

A condition of lymph fluid trapped in interstitial tissue, it can be due either to a deep chronic circulatory disorder (weak heart and pulmonary function) or weak kidney function (poor excretion of excess water). Contributing factors may be the adrenals and parathyroid glands (help in water balance) and blocked or under-functioning lymph transport. In cardiac oedema, the oedema will be 'pitted', i.e. when pressed the skin will stay sunken for some time, showing compromise of the heart, kidneys and circulatory systems.

Reflexes: heart, liver, lymph, kidneys, adrenal glands, parathyroids.

Swollen ankles

Many people suffer from swollen ankles when standing for long periods, or travelling on aircraft or sitting a long time, or in very hot weather. These transient states of oedema can be greatly helped.

Reflexes: lymph with kidr
for ADH, adrenal glands.

Sudden swelling

In cases of sudden swelling
they control the sodium-po
lymphatic tissue will swell
and/or lymph vessels will b
than normal tissue, thus in
temporarily or permanentl

Reflexes: the site of the tr
reflexes, possible cross refl

Auxiliary treatment: clea
salt.

Cellulite

A condition where lymph is congested (fluid retention) in connective tissue, and fat cells become harder. The skin has an 'orange peel' or dimpled appearance.

Reflexes: lymph and eliminative channels, adrenal glands, circulation.

Cellulitis

Skin and connective tissue become the focus for bacterial infection causing fever, swelling, inflammation and pain. If this spreads to the blood vessels it can lead to more serious septicaemia so should be referred to a GP.

Reflexes: lymph and eliminative reflexes plus adrenals.

Auxiliary treatment: manual lymph drainage. For the cellulite, advise a cleansing diet and exercise and massage. For cellulitis, advise as for any infection: rest, fasting, herbal antibiotics, aromatic teas.

Sprains and strains

See also Oedema (above) *and also refer to* musculo-skeletal conditions (page 242).

Reflexes: immediately the cross reflex for the affected joint or muscle. If the injury is not on the feet itself, the reflex on the foot for that particular area, for example knee reflex for knee injury. Lymphatic system. **Back-up reflexes**: adrenal and kidneys, as well as stress. Reflexology can speed recovery and healing.

Wounds, surgery, trauma

Whenever the skin is pierced and the underlying tissues are cut, lymph vessels are also cut, and traumatised. The body's defence mechanisms come into play, in which the lymph plays a vital part. Giving reflexology both before and after surgery greatly improves the outcome.

Reflexes: lymphatic system, spleen, immune system, adrenals, stress reflexes.

Auxiliary: Star of Bethlehem Bach flower remedy, arnica in the form of homeopathic tablets, cream or in the form of a tincture to add to bathing water.

Fatigue

See also Endocrine system (pages 221 and 223).

Fatigue can be caused by multiple factors and come under several systems. Among these factors are: excessive activity or overwork, under-activity, malnutrition, circulatory problems of blood and lymph, respiratory disturbance, infections – including recent acute ones and low-grade viral infections, nervous exhaustion/stress/depression, endocrine disturbances, even poor posture. It is extremely important that you explore all these possibilities and work the corresponding reflexes.

Reflexes: lymphatic system in all cases of fatigue. **Back-up reflexes**: endocrine glands, digestive system, nervous system, stress reflexes, as indicated and the other eliminative channels.

HIV-AIDS

See also Endocrine system (page 221).

Current research in the United States is showing that those HIV patients who engage in complementary therapies have a longer survival rate and/or show a reduction in negative symptoms than those who use only orthodox medical treatment. Appropriate complementary treatments include the use of herbs and nutritional supplements, acupuncture, stress management and energy conservation, and lifestyle changes. Consider a multi-disciplinary approach and refer to other practitioners and medical physicians.

Reflexology can play a vital role in such treatments. The most obvious benefits derive from its promotion of deep relaxation, recovery from stress, and reflexology's beneficial effect on the lymphatic-endocrine-immune system. Of course, in such a condition every system needs attention, including digestive, respiratory and the eliminative channels. However, do not expect quick results, work carefully and gradually, adapting the technique to the client's state of mind and body, for the best results.

Conditions involving imbalance of the urinary system

Lower back pain

Remarkable as it may seem, this can be due to irritation or inflammation of the kidneys which affects the surrounding tissues. So it is always worth asking if there is a history of kidney weakness, or infection. Also in traditional Chinese medicine, the kidneys influence the lower body and legs. Remember their anatomical position in the body. Osteopaths say that after treatment, kidneys that have been held high because of back muscle tension can actually 'drop' down to a more normal position.

Reflexes: kidneys, adrenal glands, spine, especially lower back.

Incontinence

This occurs most often either in childhood or in older age, but can also be a result of pregnancy and childbirth or operations which leave the bladder muscles weakened, and result in 'stress incontinence'. It can also be a symptom of renal disease and prostate problems, cystitis, irritable bladder syndrome, or the result of diuretic drugs for heart disease/hypertension.

Reflexes: urinary system, stress, glands. For sphincter muscle weakness, work the adrenals, the pelvic muscle reflexes (ankle areas), and in women include the reproductive areas.

Auxiliary treatment: Bach flower remedies, mild nervine/calming herb teas such as chamomile. Pelvic floor exercises. Avoid tea, coffee, alcohol.

Cystitis

An acute bacterial infection of the bladder which can be extremely painful; there is a burning sensation on passing urine. The danger is that it may spread further up and into the kidneys themselves but this is not usual.

Reflexes: urinary, immune system, lymphatic and other eliminative channels, endocrine glands, especially adrenals.

Auxiliary treatment: cut out all tea and coffee. Adopt an alkaline or cleansing diet. At the acute stage, recommend the client drinks increased amounts of water, at least 275ml (½ pt) of cold water or barley water every 20 minutes until the crisis passes. Thereafter, 3 litres (5 pints) a day until urine is normal. Cranberry juice, aduki bean and mung beans are helpful. Ensure adequate rest and examine any stress factors in the life. Use cotton underwear only (or go without any), washed only in mild soap, not biological detergent.

Renal stones, renal colic

Stones are accretions of calcium and other salts in one or both kidneys; they may be associated with gout, parathyroid problems or kidney disease. If a stone passes out of the kidney but lodges in the ureter, great pain or colic is caused.

Reflexes: kidney and bladder, diaphragm/solar plexus. **Back-up reflexes**: diaphragm, parathyroids, stress.

Auxiliary treatment: acute: hot water bottle or ice pack locally. Cleansing diet. Avoid tea, coffee, alcohol. Increase fluid intake.

Nephritis or Bright's disease

Inflammation of the glomeruli, the tiny filters in the kidneys, causing red blood cells and protein to leak into urine. Can lead to anaemia, high blood pressure or renal failure if waste products accumulate as a result.

Reflexes: kidneys-bladder, adrenals. **Back-up reflexes**: immune system, lymphatics, renal nerves, stress reflexes.

Auxiliary treatment: nephritis is best referred to a doctor or medical herbalist but reflexology can definitely help by supporting and enhancing the body's healing efforts. Advise a cleansing diet avoiding tea, coffee, alcohol; rest, and stress reduction exercises.

Gout

Painful swelling and inflammation of the big toe, elbow, knuckles or knee. Caused by the build-up of urates or uric acid crystals around the joint. It is a form of arthritis. The kidneys should be excreting the urates, but if for some reason they fall behind, or too much is created in the body for them to cope with, the uric acid crystals accumulate in spaces between joints (or even in the kidneys themselves). Can be the result of diet, or genetic factors, but also from leukaemia and psoriasis which have weakened the kidneys. Repeated episodes of gout should be referred for medical investigation for raised white blood cell count (leukaemia). Check the case history, ask about parents' history.

Reflexes: kidneys, adrenal glands, diaphragm/solar plexus, eliminative channels. **Back-up reflexes**: knee, stress.

Auxiliary treatment: cleansing diet, alkaline diet, and avoid coffee, tea, alcohol and meat especially.

Conditions involving imbalances of the digestive system

Ulcers

Pain and burning sensations in the chest or upper abdomen, lasting up to three hours, with indigestion, nausea, or vomiting are symptoms. Very related to stress, especially emotions of frustration and anger. Recent research suggests it may be caused by a bacteria (Helicobacter pylori) in the lining of the stomach. Normally treated medically with drugs Zantac or Tagamet which inhibits gastric acid production, or now with antibiotics. Reflexology can surely help here.

Reflexes: stomach, diaphragm, duodenum, nerves to stomach, small and large intestines. **Back-up reflexes**: stress, immune system.

Auxiliary treatment: Bach flower remedies. Eat only small amounts at a time, chewing thoroughly. Take slippery elm powder. Cleansing diet. Avoid rich, sugary, fatty or spicy foods.

Appendicitis

Inflammation of the lymphoid tissue in the appendix, which may become perforated and abscessed; signs are colicky pain around or below the navel, nausea or vomiting, possibly dysuria (painful urination), if the appendix lies over the urethra, slight fever and furred tongue with foul breath. If or when pain localises at McBurney's point (halfway between navel and right iliac crest), it causes extreme pain on pressure. If abscessed, the appendix is drained or removed. While still in the 'grumbling appendix' stage (recurrent bouts of the above symptoms) reflexology can definitely help heal the area, preventing it reaching the perforated stage, and helping relieve pain. Post-surgery, reflexology treatment is very beneficial in promoting healing and removing the imbalances which caused it in the first place.

Reflexes: ileo-caecal valve, diaphragm, lymph, pelvic region. **Back-up reflexes**: adrenal and stress reflexes. Points will be painful so sensitive handling is required.

Auxiliary treatment: look for factors causing lymph tissue to become congested – toxicity due to diet, or general lymphatic congestion.

Candida albicans/candidiasis

See also Immune system (page 221).

This is a relatively recently recognised condition, although naturopaths, iridologists, and Ayurvedic medicine have long known and treated conditions of toxicity in the colon. Today candida refers to a yeast or fungus infection of the small intestine. It is said that all of us have some candida but that in some, it starts to grow and get out of control producing a large number and variety of symptoms. Often this increase is brought on by poor diet, stress or the repeated use of antibiotics, which weaken the immune system and destroy the 'friendly' bacteria which inhabit the gut, thus leaving the field free for the candida to proliferate. Symptoms include: genital and oral thrush, general fatigue, headaches, migraines, joint pains, vaginitis, indigestion, diarrhoea, constipation, abdominal distention, food allergies, depression, irritability, memory lapse, concentration loss, mouth ulcers.

Reflexes: stomach, liver, gall bladder, pancreas, intestines, especially ileo-caecal valve, sigmoid rectum, and anus. **Back-up reflexes**: stress reflexes, immune reflexes. Accompany with a strict cleansing diet to have good effects.

Auxiliary treatment: anti-candida diet restricting all sugars, alcohol, vinegar, any food containing moulds, certain fruits, meat, eggs, dairy products. Kitcheree. Flower remedies.

Constipation

Lack of regular, daily passing of stools. Recently we have avoided paying much attention to constipation in reaction to the obsession about it in Victorian times. But the fact is that all cultures recognise the importance of regular evacuation of stools as part of keeping the internal environment of the body clean. Constipation equates to not removing your kitchen waste regularly, resulting in an environment of putrefaction, fermentation, literally an attraction for 'bugs'. Even medical science is beginning to pay more attention: recent research shows women who suffer from constipation, defined as delayed transit time of the contents of the colon, are more likely to have gallstones. Toxins can accumulate then seep out through the bowel wall to re-enter the blood and be circulated around the body. They will accumulate in the body's weakest spots and become the foundation for many conditions. This is why people who go on a cleansing diet, fast or cleanse the colon with reflexology or herbs find a marked reduction in or disappearance in their symptoms in many conditions – anything from arthritis, to varicose veins, to headaches, to depression. In holistic terms, constipation represents an excess of the earth element, possibly due to fear.

Reflexes: stomach, liver-gall bladder, pancreas, intestines, especially ileo-caecal valve, sigmoid rectum, and anus. 'Chronic' area at the back of the Achilles tendon. **Back-up reflexes**: diaphragm, adrenal, spinal nerves to the area.

Auxiliary treatment: liver cleanse, cleansing diet or fast, then a healthy diet, with plenty of liquids, fresh fruit and vegetables, and exercise. Examine such factors as emotional 'holding'.

Chron's Disease
Cause unknown, inflammation of the ileum where it merges with the large intestine, causing severe cramping pains after eating, diarrhoea, weakness and sometimes fever. Can become serious, leading to anaemia, or peritonitis and, rarely, provoke cancer. Recurs, though maybe with months or years between bouts. After each episode, tissues heal but may scar over, narrowing the lumen and thus interfering with absorption of nutrients and creating difficulty with stools.

Reflexes: ileo-caecal valve, whole intestines, stomach, liver-gall bladder, pancreas. Feet may be very tender! Patient may be very afraid of any pain. Don't be in a hurry, work gradually, gently. **Back-up reflexes**: diaphragm, adrenal, spinal nerves to area, stress reflexes, immune reflexes.

Auxiliary treatment: as for constipation (facing page). Relaxation and stress reduction techniques. Self-massage of the abdomen.

Colitis, irritable bowel syndrome, nervous diarrhoea
Alternating diarrhoea and constipation with cramping pains in the lower abdomen, possibly pain on defecating. Muscle action may be uncoordinated or spasmodic. Usually due to stress factors, possibly phobias, but may also be due to dietary allergies, candidiasis, spinal misalignments, excessive use of laxatives or even parasites in the colon.

Reflexes: digestive tract, especially liver-gall bladder, ileum and colon; stress reflexes. **Back-up reflexes**: spinal nerves to area, immune reflexes.

Auxiliary treatment: cleansing diet, slippery elm powder, identify and reduce/relieve stress factors in life, relaxation and breathing exercises. Referral to osteopath, chiropractor, herbalist, if indicated.

Coeliac disease
Malabsorption and failure to thrive caused by allergy to gluten in some grains which cause the villi in the small intestine to atrophy and thus limit absorption. First identified in infants after weaning but now appearing also in adults with symptoms of anaemia and emaciation, distended abdomen, itching, abdominal pains, diarrhoea-constipation.

Reflexes: stomach, digestive tract, especially small intestines. **Back-up reflexes**: spinal nerves to the area, adrenal and all glands, stress and immune reflexes.

Auxiliary treatment: abstain from foods containing gluten. Cleansing diet.

Diverticulitis

Inflammation of diverticuli or pockets which have formed in the bowel wall, harbouring toxins. These become prone to infection, (inflammation). Symptoms include cramps in lower, left abdomen, fever, nausea. There is the risk of peritonitis.

Reflexes: large intestines, adrenal, diaphragm. **Back-up reflexes**: entire digestive tract, glands, spinal nerves to area, liver-gall bladder, immune reflexes.

Auxiliary treatment: cleansing diet, high fibre diet. Liver cleanse.

Flatulence

Accumulation of gas in the digestive tract. Can be due to poor food, poor digestion.

Reflexes: stomach, liver-gall bladder, pancreas, intestines. **Back-up reflexes**: diaphragm, spinal nerves to area.

Auxiliary treatment: improve diet; cook with carminatives such as fennel, cumin, dill, ginger. Eat slowly, taking small bites. Relax before and after eating. Chew thoroughly. Cleansing diet and/or brief fast to cleanse colon; enemas.

Gastro-enteritis (food poisoning)

Acute, bacterial infection of the digestive tract producing symptoms such as mild fever, diarrhoea, possible vomiting as the body tries to cleanse itself of the bacteria.

Reflexes: stomach, liver-gall bladder, small and large intestines. **Back-up reflexes**: diaphragm, stress-immune-lymphatic system.

Auxiliary treatment: rest, water to restore fluids, a brief fast will help cleanse the system.

Haemorrhoids

Dilated blood vessels inside or at the opening of the anus, causing swelling with irritation, itching, and sometimes bleeding. Can become chronic and strangulated and require an operation. Cause is usually constipation with straining to pass stools, but can happen even in those who evacuate regularly; constant flatulence may be putting undue pressure on the tissues. Other causes can be persistent coughing, standing for long periods, laxatives, sitting on cold surfaces and travelling long distances sitting. Many women develop them in pregnancy or after childbirth, due to pressure on the area.

Reflexes: stomach, liver-gall bladder, pancreas, intestines, ileo-caecal valve, sigmoid, rectum, anus, chronic area at the back of the Achilles tendon. **Back-up reflexes**: diaphragm, adrenal glands.

Auxiliary treatment: as above for constipation, externally apply comfrey or chickweed ointment. Head stands, shoulder stands/ tip-up methods. Warm Epsom salts baths.

Hiatus hernia

Weakness of the tissue surrounding the hiatus – the hole in the diaphragm through which the oesophagus passes. This allows the stomach to herniate (protrude) up into the diaphragm, putting pressure on the oesophageal valve and gradually weakening it. This then allows acids from the stomach to reflux into the oesophagus causing a burning pain.

Reflexes: stomach, oesophagus. **Back-up reflexes**: stomach nerves, diaphragm, stress reflexes – especially adrenal glands.

Auxiliary treatment: eat slowly, and never late at night. Raise the head of the bed, if possible. Avoid alcohol and smoking.

Heartburn, acid indigestion

Minor stomach/or lower chest pain, belching, discomfort, hiccups after eating. Can be caused by a number of factors, but especially look at the environment around meal times: the style of eating (too fast, not chewed, too large amounts/bites, eating in front of the television). Other provokers include stress, allergies, hypoglycaemia, candidiasis, peptic ulcers, gallstones, pancreas problems and even cancer. If there are sudden changes or the condition is not related to the first factors, refer the client to a doctor for examination.

Reflexes: stomach, oesophagus, diaphragm. **Back-up reflexes**: nerves to stomach, adrenal and stress reflexes.

Auxiliary treatment: relaxation/meditation before eating. Eating in small bites, smaller amounts, more often; chew thoroughly. Relax after eating. No late night eating; avoid tea, coffee, alcohol, smoking. Bach flower remedies to calm, balance mental sphere.

Gallstones

Solidification of various substances in bile such as calcium and cholesterol. May be present but unknown/unfelt and pass without notice. But if a stone becomes trapped as it passes out, it causes swelling with build-up of bile in the gall bladder. Therefore fats pass into the small intestine undigested, with pain, nausea, vomiting and discomfort after eating fatty foods. Constipation may be a sign of poor gall bladder function or stones. A hypo-thyroid condition with a sluggish metabolism may be a factor. A more severe condition is cholecystis, an acute condition of inflammation of the gall bladder and biliary colic with intense pain in the upper right abdomen, or between the shoulders, nausea, and vomiting. This in turn may trigger jaundice or peritonitis. Orthodox medicine removes stones by surgery or laser treatment. Over two or three weeks, reflexology will gradually help the bile duct to dilate. If or when the client experiences sharp cutting pains, stop treatment and allow nature to proceed unaided. Resume treatment once the pain has stopped.

Reflexes: gall bladder, liver, entire digestive tract. **Back-up reflexes**: thyroid, adrenal, diaphragm, spinal nerves to organs.

Auxiliary treatment: liver cleanse. Cleansing diet, then healthy diet. Identification of emotional factors – anger, frustration, resentment, jealousy. Bach flower remedies. Exercise.

Hepatitis

Infection and inflammation of the liver caused by Hepatitis A or B virus, glandular fever virus, yellow fever, alcohol and certain drugs. May be acute or chronic. Medical attention should be sought.

Reflexes: liver, gall bladder, glands and immune system. Spinal nerves to area. Immune reflexes, stress reflexes. **Back-up reflexes**: elimination channel reflexes.

Auxiliary treatment: rest and cleansing diet, then a healthy diet. When well and strong, liver cleanse may be taken.

Hypoglycaemia

see under Endocrine system (page 221)

Jaundice

A condition of the liver producing a yellowing of the skin and sclera (coating of the eyeball), stools turn grey and chalky. Several reasons may be responsible such as gallstones, drugs (for example, paracetamol, anabolic steroids, Valium, oral contraceptives) all of which must be processed and detoxified by the liver. May worsen into hepatitis.

Reflexes: liver-gall bladder, entire digestive tract, glands and immune system, stress reflexes. **Back-up reflexes**: according to other factors identified.

Auxiliary treatment: cleansing diet, then healthy wholefood diet, avoid drugs if possible. After condition eases, may cleanse with liver cleanse.

Eating disorders

These include bulimia or compulsive overeating, anorexia or compulsive undereating and wasting. There are complex psychological factors causing these problems and expert help should be sought. Reflexology can play an important part by helping to balance the glandular system, inducing relaxation, relieving stress and nourishing self-esteem via the sense of touch.

Reflexes: diaphragm, stomach and digestive tract, spinal nerves, glands and endocrine system. **Back-up reflexes**: stress reflexes.

Conditions involving imbalance of the reproductive system

Amenorrhea

Temporary or permanent absence of menstrual periods. Termed 'primary' when the menarche is delayed at puberty, and 'secondary' when periods have started then later stopped. Secondary may be due to several factors including anorexia or extreme weight loss, extreme exercise, stress, coming off the pill, and, rarely, displacement of the uterus.

Reflexes: ovaries, uterus, chronic reflex of Achilles tendon, all glands, spinal nerves to reproductive organs and glands. **Back-up reflexes**: stress reflexes, immune reflexes, diaphragm/solar plexus.

Auxiliary treatment: counselling; flower remedies, dietary/food therapy; appropriate exercise (yoga or t'ai chi); relaxation and breathing.

Dysmenorrhea
Painful periods. Most women suffer some discomfort during the first day or two of the period. But many women suffer more extreme cramping pains and malaise, with possible nausea or vomiting. Some women become extremely fearful and anxious. Sometimes this occurs after coming off the pill, or using an IUD. It is important to note that if periods suddenly become painful after several years of otherwise normal periods, then investigate for presence of fibroids, endometriosis, or PID (pelvic inflammatory disease). Refer the client to their GP but you may continue with reflexology.

Reflexes: ovaries, uterus, chronic uterus, endocrine glands, spinal nerves. **Back-up reflexes**: diaphragm/solar plexus, stress reflexes.

Auxiliary treatment: Bach flower remedies, t'ai chi, yoga postures, relaxation and breathing.

Menorrhagia
Heavy periods with profuse bleeding, flooding, discharge of clots, bleeding lasting more than seven days. In general, it is due to hormonal imbalances. Offering constitutional treatment and education to balance this as much as possible is therefore the best approach. Another possibility is that the body is using the menses as a means of eliminating excess toxicity if others are blocked or congested. Reflexology can of course play a valuable part, helping to cleanse the body and balance the hormonal system. Other causes may be: IUD, fibroids or endometriosis, PID. If a period is suddenly heavy and clotty after recent intercourse, it may be an early, undetected miscarriage. These possibilities need to be checked and appropriate referrals made. Repeated heavy periods can cause anaemia, and fatigue with so much loss of blood.

Reflexes: uterus, ovaries, all glands, spinal nerves, eliminative channels, liver. **Back-up reflexes**: diaphragm/solar plexus, immune system, stress reflexes.

Auxiliary treatment: cleansing diet and wholefood diet rich in iron, avoiding heating spices and greasy foods; natural iron supplements; liver cleanse and diet; flower remedies to balance constitution; yoga, t'ai chi.

Depression
This seems to affect women a little more than men. In women it can be related to hormonal imbalance, fatigue or congestion associated with periods. *See also under* Nervous system (page 217). **Reflexes**: reproductive organs, liver. nerves, diaphragm/solar plexus, stress.

Endometriosis
A condition in which fragments of the endometrium (womb lining) migrate to the fallopian tubes, ovaries, vagina and even intestines. Here they are still sensitive to hormone messages and so engorge every month

with blood and irritate and scar surrounding tissue. Symptoms include heavy periods, dragging period pains worse towards the end of the period, painful intercourse. Orthodox treatment is to prescribe the contraceptive pill or drugs to inhibit ovulation temporarily to allow the body time to re-absorb the tissue; surgical removal of fragments; hysterectomy. It has been noted that this condition may be more common in high-achieving, working women, which suggests a possible inner conflict over roles in certain women, a subject which may be worth exploring with the client.

Reflexes: uterus, ovaries, fallopian tubes, intestines, pelvic region in general (may be tender, touch gently), all glands, spinal nerves, liver, eliminative channels. **Back-up reflexes**: diaphragm/solar plexus, stress.

Auxiliary treatment: cleansing diet, wholefood diet. Flower remedies, yoga postures, t'ai chi. Relaxation and breathing. Visualisations.

Swollen breasts, lumps

Swollen, tender breasts occur with the hormonal cycle and with PMS, part of the general fluid congestion built up by some women before a period. Treat this as part of PMS below. Breast lumps may be created by the formation of cysts (a fluid-filled sac of tissue), by fibro-adenosis (thickening of the lactic tissue), which can change to a benign growth or to a malignant growth. If the patient notices any change in nipple shape, skin colour or texture, the 'hang' of the breasts, or any hard or tender areas that do not move, refer to a GP immediately.

Reflexes: breasts, all lymphatics, ovaries and all endocrine glands especially pituitary, urinary system. **Back-up reflexes**: other eliminative channels and the liver.

Auxiliary treatment: cleansing diet, adequate rest and exercise. Avoid caffeine, chocolate.

PMS (Pre-menstrual syndrome or tension)

This is really a group of symptoms which affect many women just before the period. They vary with the individual but include: swollen or tender breasts, fluid retention, weight gain, abdominal bloating, headaches, mood swings, anxiety, back pain, nausea, fatigue, irritability. Depression may be a predisposing factor. Holistically speaking, PMS reflects not only imbalances in the hormonal system (physical level) but also suggests the mental-emotional aspect of the woman's life may not be happy. In fact the two things cannot be totally separated, as hormonal imbalances can produce emotional imbalances and vice versa. It is important to discuss with the woman relevant aspects of her life and to try to determine her sense of self-esteem. For example, does she feel generally empowered in her life or conversely, is she overly controlling? As said before, symptoms are the body's way of communicating that all is not well, so they should be paid attention to and not merely dismissed as an inevitable part of being a woman. The time around the period is like a moment of truth; things which bother us but which can be hidden other times, now make themselves felt! The time between ovulation and the period (progesterone phase) is an inward phase, when, by tuning in to our inner feelings and experiences, we can gain deeper understanding about ourselves and others in our lives. Reflexology can definitely help many women by allowing them the space to be with themselves, giving them permission to focus on themselves for a change, as well as by stimulating the body to balance endocrine secretions.

Reflexes: endocrine system and reproductive systems, the spinal column for nerve supply, the eliminative channels, the abdominal and pelvic areas. **Back-up reflexes**: stress and diaphragm/solar plexus.

Auxiliary treatment: flower remedies, cleansing diet, wholefood diet low in fats (fat increases blood levels of oestrogen), cut out caffeine, alcohol, smoking. Relaxation and breathing exercises. Evening primrose oil, star flower or flaxseed oil; supplements such as Vitamin B complex, calcium and magnesium. Increase dietary intake of soya products and pulses, fresh fruits and vegetables; these all contain isoflavones which regulate oestrogen levels.

Ovarian cysts, polyps

Fluid-filled tissue on or around the ovaries. Invisible and symptomless unless they grow large enough to bear down on the bladder or show as swelling. The menstrual cycle may be affected, becoming irregular. They are not dangerous except for risk that if they burst peritonitis will result. This is an example of the body trying to contain and isolate morbid matter which it cannot otherwise eliminate.

Reflexes: ovaries, uterus and pelvic region, spinal nerves to the reproductive area, all lymphatics, circulation, immune system, eliminative channels.

Auxiliary treatment: flower remedies. Cleansing diet, wholefood diet. Exercise, relaxation, visualisations.

Fibroids

Non-cancerous growths in or on the uterus; rather common in women between 30 and 50. Small ones are symptomless and tend to disappear after age of 45 with the menopause but larger ones provoke heavy, prolonged and very painful periods, with pain on intercourse, and possibly cystitis if they press on the bladder. If a large one becomes twisted it causes severe lower abdominal pain. Orthodox treatment is a D&C (dilation and curettage) and possibly hysterectomy.

Reflexes: uterus, ovaries, and all glands, eliminative channels. **Back-up reflexes**: chronic uterus reflex, stress reflexes, spinal reflexes to area.

Auxiliary treatment: flower remedies. Cleansing diet, then wholefood diet high in fibre, and low in animal fats and animal protein.

Infertility

This is a complex condition, factors will vary with each client, and a multi-dimensional approach is needed. Reflexology can definitely be a valuable part of a programme to increase fertility in both women and men. It will improve all body functions and reduce the effects of the stress such a condition creates in the person's life.

Reflexes: uterus/prostate, ovaries/testes, all endocrine glands, including pituitary. Spinal nerves, especially to glands and uterus. Diaphragm and stress reflexes.

Auxiliary treatments: flower remedies, cleansing diet, then wholefood diet, relaxation and exercise. Visualisations. Advise organic foods only, Vitamin B12, folic acid, magnesium, zinc, anti-oxidants such as Vitamin E, selenium. Referral to a nutritionist

Prostate problems

Benign Prostate Hypertrophy (BPH) has become quite common in men over 40. It is a benign swelling of the prostate, putting pressure on the bladder, with corresponding symptoms of frequent nocturnal urination, sudden urges to urinate but with slow or hesitant stream, dribbling of urine, maybe blood in urine, frequent need to urinate. In addition to swelling, the gland tissues change, becoming less elastic, perhaps developing small nodules. To compensate, the bladder muscles become stronger to keep the urethra open. It is possible that the bladder will not empty fully leaving residual urine which becomes the focus for bladder and possibly kidney infection. Cause is 'unknown' but involves such things as hormone imbalance associated with ageing, pesticide or chemical residue exposure (concentrates androgens in the prostate which cause over-production of cells).

Reflexes: prostate, testes, vas deferens; all glands. Lower spine, chronic area of the Achilles tendon.

Auxiliary treatment: organic food, cleansing diet, wholefood diet. Evening primrose oil, starflower and flaxseed oils, zinc.

Rites of passage

These are transitional periods in life when we move from one stage to another through changes initiated by the endocrine system. In more traditional societies these are marked by special ceremonies of celebration and welcoming into the company of those in the next stage. Such traditions give a public acknowledgement that the person is facing new challenges and responsibilities and is now in a different relationship with themselves and the community, with different rights and responsibilities. Unfortunately, Western society has lost many of these traditions, though remnants remain. As a result, some people suffer from the stress such change places on them or from confusion over their new roles and responsibilities. This can have an effect on their health. At the same time, experience of these transitions can also be affected by the body's state of health. A body relatively free of toxicity and with a free movement of energy through it will pass through such transitions more easily. Reflexology can play an important role here. In the first instance, it helps to balance hormonal activity, keep the body free of toxins and stagnation and provide relaxation and stress recovery. In the second it can provide that therapeutic space in which the person can reflect on, sift through and integrate the new circumstances.

Puberty

We all pay lip service to the fact that our teenagers are feeling the effects of hormonal changes, effects which can influence their behaviours. Yet we do little to help them pass through this transition as smoothly as possible. What can we do? In addition to reflexology treatments, we can guide them towards a healthier diet (almost impossible with a teenager but try), encourage them to take regular exercise they enjoy (girls are especially prone to give up exercise/sports during this stage) and provide positive experiences for them away from constant media stimulation.

Reflexes: reproductive areas, spinal nerves, all glands, diaphragm/solar plexus, eliminative channels, liver.

Auxiliary treatment: flower remedies, cleansing and wholefood diet, exercise, especially yoga, t'ai chi.

Conception

Both parents could do their children a world of good by preparing themselves not only for childbirth but for conception itself. Bringing the body to its optimum state of health, cleansing it of congestions, improving hormonal and reproductive function, and creating a calm, alert mental and emotional atmosphere are the best means to give the child the best chance in life right from the start. Reflexology can play an important part in such an approach.

Reflexes: eliminative channels, all glands, nerves.

Pregnancy and childbirth

Reflexology is generally safe for pregnancy although there are exceptions and cautions to be observed as discussed in Chapter 3. Many practitioners would disagree and choose not to treat duing this time. Please see Chapter 9 for information. Pregnancy is not the time to be treating specific conditions (except the diaphragm for nausea perhaps), nor to be encouraging cleansing and elimination. (The time to do this is before conception.) But a general whole-body treatment will help relax the mother, maintain her general state of health and send positive vibrations of care to the baby. A study has shown that women receiving reflexology have shorter and more comfortable labours.

In the last two weeks, reflexology treatments can help prepare for the birth, more attention can now be given to the uterus and breast areas, and adrenals. General relaxation should still be the goal.

For childbirth, reflexology can be used to help stimulate contractions if labour is delayed. Treat the uterus and chronic uterus reflexes plus the pituitary to stimulate release of labour-commencing hormone. During labour, if the mother desires it, treat the spine, especially mid and lower back, to relieve back pain, and the diaphragm/solar plexus to help relaxation and minimise anxiety. General relaxation techniques, and effleurage do help.

Post-partum

Follow the birth with a series of treatments to help normalise the body, especially hormone balance, and tonify the muscles again. This will help prevent post-natal depression and give support to the mother who is doing so much for the baby. Many women suffer severe depression after childbirth due to hormonal imbalances. The reason for the feelings of depression, possibly of indifference toward the baby, often goes unrecognised and the women who could be helped are not. Read *Depression After Childbirth* by Katharina Dalton.

Reflexes: endocrine and reproductive, adrenals, general relaxation.

Menopause

Unfortunately, for women in the West, this has become a time fraught with worries and discomforts. At last a lot more attention is being paid openly to the menopause and we are learning more about how to minimise its discomforts – but hormone replacement therapy (HRT) is not the only relief available. Reflexology can help tremendously to make this transition phase as smooth as possible, helping to balance hormones and relieve symptoms of depression, anxiety, headaches, mood swings, loss of self-confidence, hot flushes, and sleep problems. Sometimes a woman's experience of the menopause reflects her experience of her menstrual cycle throughout her life. If imbalances have been present before, and not addressed and resolved, she will experience yet more imbalance during the menopause.

Remember too, that this genuine time of transition is a turning point where roles should be re-evaluated or redefined and questioned, and new ones found. All this may be uncomfortable, change usually is, but making it a positive transition to the next phase of life will mean a healthier life in the future. Many factors can affect the experience and each woman must be understood and treated individually. Sensitivity is important with emphasis on encouraging the woman's own sense of self-esteem and self-confidence. Educate yourself as much as possible on this topic.

Reflexes: endocrine, reproductive, stress, spinal nerves. **Back-up reflexes**: liver, chronic uterus area, eliminative channels.

Male menopause

Some say that men pass through their own hormonal changes only these are much less obvious. We have seen above (page 240) that BPH is probably or partly due to hormonal changes. Certainly around the late forties and early fifties, many men go through a 'mid-life crisis', becoming anxious or uncomfortable with their roles and responsibilities in life. This can be good if it leads to positive questioning and a re-evaluation of where they are and where they are going. It's a time to get rid of a lot of excess baggage from the past, and prepare for the next phase of life. Unfortunately, many men seem to find this such a time of anxiety that instead of turning within and working with it, they look outside themselves for security, or challenge themselves in new or impossible ways in order to prove themselves still virile.

A better way to pass through is to undertake a programme of cleansing and tonification aided and guided by reflexology. Diet, exercise, flower remedies, yoga, t'ai chi should be a part of this programme.

Reflexes: same as for women.

Conditions of imbalance in the musculo-skeletal system

Arthritis, osteo-

Osteo-arthritis affects the cartilage and lubricating fluid covering articulating surfaces causing underlying bone to thicken and distort. This restricts joint movement, provokes episodes of pain, swelling and inflammation. Usually affects load bearing joints but not always. Causes may be overuse, injury, age, diet (one high in animal protein and fats creates excess acidity which can be associated with arthritis), calcium metabolism (calcium is not kept in solution but gets deposited in weak areas), toxins from the colon which settle in a weak joint causing inflammation. Circulation to the area is impeded, thus less waste is removed (cleansing), and cell renewal is affected (nutrition). Psychologically this can reflect 'armouring', or inflexibility.

Reflexes: affected area or cross reflex, spine, parathyroids (calcium metabolism), adrenal (mineral metabolism, natural cortisone).
Back-up reflexes: liver, kidneys, large intestine and all eliminative channels, diaphragm/solar plexus.

Auxiliary treatment: flower remedies; hot-cold hydrotherapy; cleansing alkaline diet, wholefood diet, Hay diet. Apple cider vinegar with honey in the morning. Epsom salts in hot baths. Keep exercising: yoga, t'ai chi, swimming. Weight-loss may be indicated, to ease stress on joints.

Arthritis, rheumatoid

An auto-immune condition in which an inflammatory response is activated by the body's own protein. Synovial fluid around joints inflames and swells causing pain. May spread to surrounding tissues, even bone, sometimes to heart and blood vessels. Repeated flare-ups gradually dry out the fluid and deteriorate joint tissue. Mainly affects smaller joints: knuckles, neck, ankles, toes, wrists, also knees.

Reflexes: specific area affected or cross reflex, spinal nerves. Diaphragm, eliminative channels, immune reflexes, stress reflexes, all glands.

Auxiliary treatment: cleansing, alkaline diet, wholefood diet, flower remedies. Moderate exercise: yoga, t'ai chi, swimming. Epsom salt baths.

Backache

This is perhaps one of the most common ailments today and can come from a variety of causes, most often muscle strain, postural imbalance (twisted pelvis, short-leg), herniated disc, trauma caused by injury or accidents, even birth trauma may set up a pattern of imbalance that will manifest later in life as backache; kidney energy imbalance can also manifest in back pains (see page 230).

Taking a careful case history and observing the posture will help you pinpoint the origin. Reflexology is effective both in relieving back pain and relaxing the muscles whose chronic tension pull discs and or other muscles out of alignment, thus allowing the spine to realign itself.

Reflexes: whole spine, necks of all toes, particular muscles, vertebrae, or nerves affected but also corresponding ones. For example, upper body imbalance may lead to low back pain so explore and treat these areas also. Shoulder, adrenal, stress reflexes. **Back-up reflexes**: diaphragm/ solar plexus. Pituitary for the release of endorphins to help with pain; shoulder, hip, knee, sciatic; chronic area of Achilles tendon.

Auxiliary treatment: flower remedies; back exercises, yoga postures.

Bunions

This accretion of extra bone usually on the medial aspect of the first metatarsal may be due to a number of factors. Shoes are often blamed, but it can also be related to posture, thyroid function, or an unnoticed injury which traumatises the area.

Reflexes: treat on and around the affected area whenever possible to increase circulation; thyroid; shoulder. **Cross reflex area**: Same point on hand.

Auxiliary treatment: rub with castor oil daily, go barefoot as often as possible. **Exercise**: Stand with feet together at heels and toes, try to move the big toes towards each other, hold 10 seconds, then relax. Repeat several times, and several times during the day. Don't let heels move apart, but keep aiming at them touching. 'Think' the toes together.

Broken bones, dislocations, sprain or strain

See also under Lymph system (page 227).

Treat the reflex if possible or, if not, the cross reflex. For example, if it's the knee, treat the elbow on the same side. Treat the adrenals and lymph reflexes.

Auxiliary treatment: Bach flower remedies, for example Star of Bethlehem for shock.

Callus and corns

Thickening of the skin on a portion of the foot.

Reflexes: soften the area first by soaking the foot. Treat around the area, gradually working up to the area itself when tolerable. These conditions can both affect and reflect imbalances in the organ reflexed to them.

Auxiliary treatment: rub with castor oil daily.

Cramp

Muscle spasm due to shortage of oxygen and build up of lactic acid. May be precipitated by prolonged sitting, standing, or lying in awkward positions, by strenuous or exceptional exercise, or by pregnancy. Some people experience more cramps as they age, perhaps due to poor diet, lack of exercise and inadequate elimination.

Reflexes: reflex for the area, spinal nerves to area, kidneys to help eliminate lactic acid, diaphragm to induce relaxation, relieve pain.

Auxiliary treatment: magnesium or magnesium tissue salt. Improve diet and absorption of nutrients.

Bursitis

Inflammation of the pads or bursa surrounding joints which buffer friction as bone moves across bone. Bursa swell and become tender and painful. Usually self-healing if allowed to rest.

Reflexes: reflexes to specific area or cross reflex. Adrenal glands, elimination channels. **Back-up reflexes**: stress reflexes, diaphragm/solar plexus.

Auxiliary treatment: rest, hot-cold hydrotherapy.

Frozen shoulder
A 'locking' of the shoulder joint and reduced mobility due to stiffness, pain and fear of pain. Causes include injury with poor healing, bouts of bursitis or tendonitis which weaken the area.

Reflexes: shoulder area, arm, neck, spinal nerves to these areas. Lymphatics, adrenal glands, diaphragm/solar plexus. **Back-up reflexes:** stress reflexes, cross reflexes of hip and leg.

Auxiliary treatment: rest, relaxation and stretching exercises, hydrotherapy.

Gout
see under Urinary system conditions (page 231).

Slipped or herniated disc
Protrusion (rupture) of a disc from between vertebrae, causing pressure on the nerves, or rupture of ligaments and thus pain. Usually affects discs in lower back. Causes include pressure to vertebrae due to postural misalignments, pressure of wear and tear, strain.

Reflexes: reflex to particular spinal vertebra and those above and below. Whole spine to attend to areas of imbalance which may be provoking a postural imbalance. **Back-up reflexes**: adrenal glands, diaphragm/solar plexus.

Auxiliary treatment: rest, lower back exercises. Referral to an osteopath, or chiropractor if necessary. Reflexology may be just as effective however. Advise regular stretching or yoga exercise. Inverted positions if possible.

Neck tension, ache
Cause probably due to postural imbalances or traumatic injury.

Reflexes: specific of area, whole spine to balance. Shoulder, all toes, diaphragm/solar plexus.

Auxiliary treatment: self-reflexology, neck exercises. Relaxation.

Whiplash
An injury to the cervical vertebrae and muscles caused by an accident, typically motoring, which throws the person back then suddenly forward.

Reflexes: big toe and all toes, along the dorsal aspect, upper back reflexes between 1st and 2nd toes, 7th cervical, whole spine. **Back-up reflexes**: diaphragm/solar plexus, adrenal glands.

Auxiliary treatment: self-reflexology, rest. Gentle neck exercises.

Ankylosis
A condition of the cartiliginous joints of the spine, or other joints, where calcification and even eventual ossification occur as cartilage is replaced by bony tissue. Other joints affected include the Achilles tendon, the plantar fascia, hips and shoulder where cartilage tendons insert into the

bone. Symptoms are stiffness and pain gradually getting worse, with fatigue and malaise. It is important to keep moving, even though stiff and painful.

Reflexes: reflexes for the specific area. Whole spine, adrenal glands. **Back-up reflexes**: eliminative channels (especially kidneys, lymphatics), parathyroids, diaphragm/solar plexus.

Auxiliary treatment: Flower remedies, cleansing, alkaline diet, wholefood diet; yoga, t'ai chi; hot and cold hydrotherapy. Referral to osteopath, chiropractor, yoga therapist.

Sciatica
See page 220.

Conditions of imbalance of the cardio-vascular system

Angina pectoris
Basically a cramp in the heart muscle due to lack of oxygen, causing a dull, tight, constricting pain in the chest or upper abdomen, usually starting below the sternum and radiating in any direction, typically to the left arm. May come on during physical and emotional stress when extra demands are made on the heart and it is not fit to deal with it. Typical provocateurs are heavy meals, smoking, walking against a cold wind. May eventually become precursor of a heart attack. Orthodox treatment may involve drugs or a by-pass operation. Reflexology may be given if the client has consulted their doctor and received written consent.

Reflexes: heart, lungs, liver, kidneys, adrenal glands, diaphragm/solar plexus, spine, especially thoracic. **Back-up reflexes**: intestines, especially duodenum, sigmoid colon.

Auxiliary treatment: flower remedies. Rest, moderate exercise – yoga, t'ai chi. Cleansing then wholefood diet (10% fat), stopping smoking, alcohol, etc. Relaxation, stretching and breathing exercises. Self-reflexology.

Aneurysm
A swelling in the wall of the aorta or other artery (cerebral, abdominal), due to weakening of the muscle wall and which, if it bursts, is potentially lethal. Normally the swelling only presses on surrounding tissue causing, if in the aorta, pain, coughing and difficulty swallowing. Surgery may be offered, but is not always feasible. May be undetected until symptoms appear, such as sudden, severe pain at back of head or chest, throbbing lumps in abdomen. Again a serious condition which should be under medical care.

Reflexes: same as for angina, brain.

Auxiliary treatment: same as for angina.

Arrhythmia

Irregular heartbeat due to sinus node malfunction, thus disrupting electrical signals which stimulate correct contraction sequences. The basis of fibrillations, tachycardia and cardiac arrest. Orthodox treatment is anti-arrhythmic drugs, anti-coagulant drugs or beta blockers, sometimes electro-shock therapy, surgery to fit an artificial pacemaker.

Reflexes: same as for Angina.

Auxiliary treatment: flower remedies for anxiety. Same as for Angina.

Coronary disease

Disease of the heart in which the arteries become narrow or blocked by atherosclerosis. Basis of angina, coronary thrombosis or heart attack.

Reflexes: same as for Angina.

Auxiliary treatment: same as for Angina.

CVA, cardio-vascular accident, apoplexy, stroke

Interruption of blood supply to the brain causing sudden loss of speech, movement, sudden heaviness in the limbs, numbness, blurred vision, confusion, dizziness or loss of consciousness. May be only short (transient ischaemic attack or TIA) or full. Basis may be a thrombosis, embolism or haemorrhage, or atherosclerosis or arteriosclerosis which block or slow down blood supply to the brain. If blood leaks out of the vessels (haemorrhage) brain cells are damaged and do not recover, though their functions may to some extent be taken over by others.

Reflexes: brain, heart, lungs, adrenal, colon, spinal nerves especially to brain, diaphragm/solar plexus, colon, kidneys and all eliminative channels.

Auxiliary treatment: same as for Angina.

Hypertension

Persistently high blood pressure. The normal range is generally between the age of the person +100 for systolic (top figure) and above 90 to 100 diastolic. Symptoms only become apparent when consistently high pressure weakens the heart and kidneys. Causative factors are diet, arteriosclerosis, stress, overweight. Secondary hypertension is when other organs or systems are compromised, for example, kidneys, endocrine (Cushing's disease, thyroidism, toxaemia of pregnancy) and thus contribute to the hypertension. Orthodox treatment is to recommend weight loss, 30% fat diet, drugs – beta blockers,diuretics, calcium antagonists and ACE inhibitors.

Reflexes: diaphragm/solar plexus heart, lungs, liver, adrenals and all glands, kidneys, spinal nerves to these organs. **Back-up reflexes**: eliminative channels.

Auxiliary treatment: same as for Angina. Cleansing vegetarian diet of 10% fat as recommended in the book *Dr Dean Ornish's Program for Reversing Heart Disease*. Liver cleanse. Cook with fresh ginger (helps prevent blood clots), take evening primrose and other essential fatty acid oils (starflower, linseed). Avoid oral contraceptives, and HRT.

Hypotension

Low blood pressure is not considered a serious condition and some people may have blood pressure below the average, which is normal for them. It can however be part of a hypo-thyroid condition, producing a low heart rate and blood pressure. See Hypo- and Hyperthyroidism (page 222).

Phlebitis, bloodclots, thrombosis

Phlebitis is inflammation of a vein, usually due to injury or infection, producing pain, itching, redness and hard swelling; common with varicose veins. Weakening of the vessel walls, and sluggish circulation allows the development of a blood clot or thrombus, which can be dangerous as it blocks circulation, especially when in an artery to the brain, lungs or heart. These conditions require medical care but once stable, reflexology may be undertaken with the doctor's written consent.

Reflexes: heart, lung, brain, leg with cross reflexes, adrenals. **Back-up reflexes**: diaphragm. For thrombosis, observe cautions (Chapter 3).

Auxiliary treatment: vitamins B6, C and E, garlic, fresh ginger in cooking. Evening primrose, flaxseed or star flower oils, lecithin.

Varicose veins

Weakening of the walls of the veins, especially in the legs, and of the valves which help send blood back up to the heart. The result is that blood pools and distends the vessels. Smaller, more superficial vessels may become twisted and purplish, eventually poorly drained skin will turn brown. The cause may be deep vein thrombosis, constipation, obesity, pregnancy, any pelvic congestion. Complications include ulceration and thrombo-phlebitis. Orthodox treatment is to remove the varicosed sections, then close them; support stockings.

Reflexes: affected area (for example legs, knees), liver and colon and entire pelvic area, heart and adrenal glands, diaphragm/solar plexus. Cross-reflex – the arm/shoulder.

Auxiliary treatment: cleansing diet, the wholefood diet, liver cleanse. Exercise and leg exercise: legs up in air, raised as much, often as possible. Hot and cold hydrotherapy, yoga, t'ai chi.

Conditions involving imbalance of the skin

As discussed previously, skin conditions, unless due to external trauma, usually reflect the state of health of internal organs and systems. Thus it is important to assess and treat the functioning of these to gain relief. The skin most typically reflects the state of the lungs, kidneys or liver.

Acne

Eruptions on the skin due to blocked sebum pores becoming inflamed, red and swollen when bacteria is attracted to the site. Cleansing the face is important, but internal causes, such as hormone adjustments in adolescence, or a poor diet (greasy foods, chocolate), or liver function can provoke an over-production of sebum. Thus the internal systems must also be addressed. Having some acne is to be expected but when it becomes persistent it is very traumatic for a young person and saps his or her self-esteem tremendously. Careful, sensitive counselling is needed.

Reflexes: endocrine glands, especially adrenal, and thyroid, pituitary, liver, kidney and all eliminative channels. Nerves to these organs and systems, diaphragm/solar plexus.

Auxiliary treatment: flower remedies. Changes in diet, relaxation and visualisation exercises. Self-reflexology.

Eczema or dermatitis

Eczema can occur in babies, in young children, teenagers or adults. It is a local inflammation of the skin with itching, redness, weeping or flaking. It may be allergy-based (especially allergy to cow's milk, or plants, metals or detergents), or related to stress. Heredity and poor diet may be factors. It often appears in those with asthma, with asthma in their family (atopic eczema) reflecting the lung-skin connection. Again, it is the body trying to eliminate toxins which are not leaving through other channels. Alternatively, it is a hyper-allergic reaction – the body is over-reacting to a substance. Orthodox treatment is anti-inflammatory steroids, with perhaps antibiotics, but this is dangerous suppression of the condition, not a resolution.

Reflexes: adrenal, diaphragm/solar plexus, all glands, especially the thyroid, liver, all eliminative channels, especially lungs, kidneys.

Auxiliary treatment: cleansing diet, wholefood diet; withdraw allergen from diet if known. Liver cleanse (if appropriate age, it is not suitable for children under 12). Calendula ointment to relieve itching. Vitamin E, EFA oils, cold pressed vegetable oils. Flower remedies to treat the mental state (fear, anxiety, shock).

Psoriasis

The epidermis produces new cells too fast for keratin (the cohesive, protective element) to form with it. Many vitamins may be lost through this overproduction. The skin area becomes a patch of flaking, raised, pink and silver colouration, though not necessarily sore or itchy. In some it becomes more chronic and systemic, affecting joints with inflammation and swelling. Some authorities think it is a metabolic incapacity to use protein, or an enzyme deficiency. Is very stressful. It is largely an inherited condition but may be triggered by a streptococcal infection, drugs, stress, or injury. Sunlight exposure benefits many sufferers.

Reflexes: diaphragm/solar plexus, liver, all glands, especially thyroid, adrenal, eliminative channels.

Auxiliary treatment: relaxation and breathing exercises, flower remedies, supplements of vitamins C, B12, E, zinc, kelp, lecithin. Soya products, folic acid.

Excessive perspiration

This may be associated with such conditions as obesity, thyrotoxicosis (thyroid problem), Hodgkin's disease, or TB. Otherwise it may be prompted by excess alcohol, or withdrawal from alcohol, vitamin B1 deficiency, anxiety, menopause, hypoglycaemia (cold sweats). In terms of traditional medicine, it reflects low levels of vital energy. Explore all of these possibilities with your patients and treat or refer accordingly.

Miscellaneous conditions of imbalance

Allergies or sensitivities

Every era seems to have its fashionable buzzword and scapegoat for all things. At the moment it seems to be 'allergy'. The allergic response is actually a natural and appropriate alarm reaction to something the body perceives as dangerous. It recognises that the agent is 'not Me' and cannot be transformed into 'part of Me', by digestion or absorption, so it reacts to the perceived danger by creating a crisis and trying to throw out the stressor agent. For example the reaction to nettles is an allergic reaction, as is the vomiting caused by eating a poisonous berry. It is part of the body's self-defence mechanism, its immunity. The problem is that today, many people's bodies seem to be perceiving things as 'dangerous' which were not in previous times. There is much food for thought in this phenomenon.

Some allergies may be started by a particular shock or trauma to the system, such as when an infant is given cow's milk or cereal protein at an age before its digestion is set up to handle it. The body copes, but the experience is stressful and may set up a situation which can trigger later in life as an allergy. Whatever the trigger, avoiding it is only the beginning of the solution. Going deeper, we realise that by allowing the body to cleanse and rebalance, it will become better balanced, perceive more accurately and respond more appropriately to threatening agents.

Reflexology can aid this process by promoting cleansing and balance in all the systems. As well as by inducing deep relaxation and a sense of safety and security.

Reflexes: for area affected, for example, lungs, sinus, eyes as well as stress, immunity, endocrine; spine for nerves to these areas; eliminative channels, diaphragm/solar plexus.

Cancer

This may be described as an immune-compromised disease because it results from the fact that defective cells, which are produced among the 500 billion new cells formed every day, escape policing by the body's immune system and begin to multiply very rapidly and uncontrollably. Eventually they can form a tumour and invade normal tissue. There are many different types and names of cancer depending on which tissues and sites are affected. There is no single known cause, although scientists are focused on researching for a viral or defective gene cause.

Natural therapists have always emphasised the weakening of the body's own vital energy due to such factors as poor diet, toxicity, environmental pollutants, stress, or emotional trauma. Often it takes a combination of many factors to weaken the immune system so much that the cancer is triggered.

Orthodox treatment involves a combination of surgery to remove the malignant tissue and an area of healthy tissue around it, radiation to destroy cancer cells themselves, steroids, and chemotherapy or cytotoxic drugs which interfere with cell reproduction and metabolism. Unfortunately, these treatments, though sometimes necessary result in even greater trauma to the organism and may compromise it further.

Leukaemia is cancer of the white blood cells. This can spread rapidly through the lymph system.

Melanoma is cancer of the skin developing from pigment cells.

Carcinoma is cancer of the skin, developing into open sores, or wart-like lumps. This can metastasise easily so early treatment is necessary.

Reflexology could not be seen as a cure for cancer, but would form part of a programme to build up the body's immune system. It can also help to ease the anxiety and trauma caused not only by having the disease but by the treatments necessary to counter it. Whether or not to treat is somewhat controversial, and will depend on many factors, such as the type of cancer and its stage. The reflexologist must examine the subject thoroughly. It can be good to give reflexology, including before and after surgery to enhance recovery, *as long as* the client is fully consulted and the physicians's written consent has been obtained.

Reflexes would be the whole foot for general relaxation, the immune reflexes and the stress reflexes. The liver and spleen may be key reflexes in all cancers. In addition, treat the reflex for the site of the cancer and all nerves serving it. Use plenty of relaxation techniques. Counselling skills will be very much needed with cancer patients.

Auxiliary treatment: visualisation exercises, yoga and t'ai chi, flower remedies.

Case histories

The following case histories are offered to help illustrate the points made about taking case histories and record keeping made in Chapter 3.

Case 1
Mr A, aged 65, semi-retired businessman

Complaint: Mr A had been having acupuncture treatment and aromatherapy regularly for several years as he was very interested in optimising his health and keeping on top of problems. He had sinus congestion for many years and often had to breathe through his mouth. He wanted to try and see if anything could be done about this.

Consultation revealed that Mr A was very keen to keep active and healthy. His diet was a healthy one and he had been jogging several miles four days a week and working out in a gym regularly for many years. He had a tendency to get swollen ankles and congestion in his ears and sinuses; these tended to be always slightly congested. His tonsils had been removed in his youth. He had suffered digestive problems in the past but had resolved these with an anti-candida programme and enzyme supplements. This was no longer a problem. He has some varicosity of the veins in the lower legs but suffers no problems from them. Recently he had started a new business and was finding it very stressful. He had begun having palpitations.

Assessment This patient has a large build of over six feet and congestive tendencies. He is perceptive and businesslike with a good sense of humour. He is so keen to keep fit and delay ageing (an important goal) that he has a tendency to over-exert himself. The stress of his business affairs probably contributed as much to his digestive upset as the candida in the intestines due to stagnation, but he had dealt with this positively. More recent stresses were contributing to his current palpitations.

First treatment

Observations: feet are large with 'spider' veins showing above the ankle. Feet turn out considerably indicating an over-contraction of the periformis muscle/loss of muscle tone in the psoas muscles.

Reflexes: significant ones found to be tender were the nose reflex of the right foot, the left lung reflex, zone two near the diaphragm line, the liver reflex. The kidney and adrenal reflexes on both feet were very tender, and the groin lymphatic reflexes. Besides being tender, the tissue of the adrenal reflexes feels congested. I hope to work out some of this by working the reflex as well as reduce tenderness.

Assessment: the reflexes confirmed the history of stress, fluid stagnation, and some congestion in the respiratory tract.

Therapeutic strategy for next treatment: to focus on the ears, nose, sinus and respiratory points and the adrenal, kidneys and lymphatic reflexes.

Recommendation: a series of four weekly treatments particularly to see if we could help the sinus condition.

Second treatment
Response: picture was somewhat confused because he came down with flu which he believes he picked up from his wife. This could have been part of a healing through which the body was ridding itself of congestion, especially as it was not a severe case however, only short term, showing his vital energy was strong. He took extra vitamin C. No change in the sinus congestion.

Assessment of response: this could have been a mild healing crises. However, the sinus congestion was not particularly improved by this acute reaction, so this is not certain. On the other hand the sinus congestion is chronic so it may take more than one eliminative episode to resolve it. His general fitness helped him have a very mild case.

Reflexes: tender reflexes were: diaphragm right foot and left, left being more tender. The ear reflex of the right foot showed tenderness on this second treatment. The kidneys and adrenals continue to be tender and adrenals to feel congested. Special attention was given to working the stress reflexes: the adrenal and other glands, the diaphragm, and the lymphatics.

Assessment: the ear reflexes are beginning to respond to treatment; they are showing tenderness.

Third treatment
Response: the ear and sinus congestion is no better, but the palpitations have completely gone and patient reports feeling much calmer.

Therapeutic strategy: same as previous treatment.

Reflexes: the left adrenal reflex is showing more acute tenderness, right is still tender and the tissues of these areas are still congested.

Fourth treatment, two weeks later
Response: Client continues to feel calmer and to have no palpitations. Feels treatment has worked very well for that problem. However he feels no change at all in the congestion in his sinus.

Therapeutic strategy: same as previous treatment.

Reflexes: the right pituitary and thyroid helper reflexes are beginning to show tenderness, indicating that energy is beginning to enliven these glands. The left adrenal is still tender, but not the kidney. The left kidney is still tender but not the left adrenal reflex. The left ear reflex, zone 3 is still tender, but less so.

Summary
This client responded well to treatment in a significant area: his palpitations and general ability to cope with stress without becoming imbalanced. His longer standing chronic condition of congesting sinus and ears had not shown significant improvement to him, although I noticed that he did not breathe through his mouth during treatments. He felt very satisfied with the treatments, although not wishing to continue

to come every week in order to attempt to resolve his sinus problem (relatively minor from his point of view; he had learned to live with it). He would return for treatment at regular intervals to maintain his health, keep on top of the stresses.

Case 2
Mrs B, 40, married, mother of three primary school aged children

Complaint: Mrs F said that her main complaint was feeling run down, generally tired often in the morning on waking but it is usually associated with the week before her period, after which energy comes back.

During the consultation, it came out that she has a possible thyroid problem, hyperactivity, that is going to be investigated by her physician, and also that three years ago she developed fibroids, which her GP recommended she not have an operation for but offered her no other treatment. Her periods are 'all over the place': heavy, long, frequent – a 24-day cycle. She has strong PMS symptoms, becoming very irritable and angry, gets headaches, constipation, bloating, fluid retention. She often skips breakfast, but otherwise has a good appetite. Currently she is finding it difficult to get to sleep and often has to wake in the night to pass urine, but resumes sleep. Her feet feel cold and her fingers often go white.

Assessment: Mrs B is under considerable stress from her internal condition but is soldiering on with her family responsibilities. Her health is undermined by fibroids for the heavy bleeding, headaches are taking their toll; she is losing blood and iron and becoming depleted. Also the imbalances may be compounded by the possible hyperactive thyroid but this is not confirmed clinically yet. She is a tall slender woman with signs of irregularity and deficiency: lack of energy, coldness, delayed or disturbed sleep.

Recommendation: six treatments at weekly intervals, then reassess.

First treatment
Observations: feet felt cool and clammy. A whole foot treatment was given.

Reflexes: left thyroid helper, left and right chronic uterus, left uterus and ovary. Right kidney, spine at T- 8,9,10. Some lumpiness was felt by the therapist in the small intestine area. At end of treatment feet were still cool though less clammy. The tender reflexes were given extra work.

Assessment: the reflexes confirmed imbalances in the reproductive area and the thyroid gland is showing some signs of imbalance.

Therapeutic strategy: thyroid and all glands, immune reflexes, kidney and reproductive reflexes. Treatment will aid circulation and relaxation.

Second treatment
Response: Mrs B noticed no change in her complaint though she felt very relaxed after the first treatment.

Reflexes: the right and left thyroid helper reflexes showed tenderness, the reproductive reflexes still tender, adrenals now showing tenderness;

this eased on working; spinal reflexes not tender. Lymphatic reflexes of the left foot were tender.

Recommendations: self-treatment to thyroid, chronic uterus and adrenal reflexes.

Third treatment
Response: Mrs B is feeling generally better, has more energy. Her period is due in about four days and she already senses that she is feeling irritable.

Observations: her feet are now warm and not clammy, even though weather is cool.

Reflexes: the right thyroid helper, uterus, ovary and chronic uterus reflexes show no tenderness this treatment. The left thyroid helper still tender but less so. The groin lymph were very tender as were the adrenals, but adrenals eased on working.

Therapeutic strategy for next treatment: as previously.

Fourth treatment
Response: her thyroid gland seems to be acting up as she is experiencing tremors in her hands. Today she has backache as she has been decorating her mother's house. Generally she is still feeling better. When her period came she had no pain, headaches or bloating beforehand, and bleeding was less heavy, though she was still was irritable.

Reflexes: gave extra treatment to spine and shoulder reflexes to relieve current symptoms. Tenderness still reduced or not present in endocrine glands, lymph and reproductive reflexes, except the left thyroid helper and left adrenal and uterus reflexes showed tenderness.

Assessment: Mrs B is improving. Her energy is better, her body temperature is better, and her periods are much less stressful, though not completely free of discomfort. Her energy has returned and she even feels well enough to help out her parents and not feel too depleted. However, her thyroid gland is still showing signs of imbalance and she will be seeing her GP about this.

Fifth treatment
Response: Mrs B feels much better overall, even though her family activities are still demanding, and is satisfied with the improvement she has made.

Specific reflexes: Tender reflexes had all but gone in all areas. Focus of work was on the lymphatic, reproductive and pelvic areas and all the glands to boost her immune system and energy and help reduce the fibroids.

Summary
The treatments have had some considerable effect on her fibroids, perhaps lessening them to a certain extent. Her ailments associated with the periods have significantly lessened and her energy has returned and she feels able to cope with the ups and downs of her life now.

Case 3
Mr C, aged 21, recently graduated in economics from university, seeking employment. Tall and medium build, dark hair.

Complaint: discharges from eyes and nose. Nasal discharge alternates between yellow and white and his throat frequently needs clearing. Discharge from eyes is worse in the morning, starts like dandruff on the lashes, then with movement a white discharge starts, then a yellow type of scab forms which he removes and then it becomes red. Some foods worsen eyes, but not carefully identified – certainly bread, possibly sugar, alcohol. He is also feeling very lethargic, lacks motivation. He had received homeopathic treatment and was recommended to take acidopholus for candida associated with lethargy, which has helped a bit. He had his appendix removed four years ago and had to go on antibiotics.

During the consultation it emerged that he had suffered from night sweats since childhood and this is still an occasional problem. He sweats very easily; his palms often sweat. His mouth is often dry. He gets cold sores a lot. He feels he has somewhat frequent urination, compared to others. He gets little exercise these days though enjoyed running at school. His bowels are usually regular once a day, except when he feels unwell as now in which case they become irregular either twice a day or not every day at all. He sleeps heavily but wakes up lethargic, legs feeling like lead and mind slow whereas at night his mind is very active. Emotionally he enjoys loving relationships with his family and friends. His diet includes a lot of fruit and vegetables, is omnivore. He drinks a lot of herbal tea.

Assessment: Mr C is a strongly motivated achieving person, but whose current pattern is one of deficiency and imbalance related to the nervous system, which he may have had a tendency towards since childhood. The deficiency is suggested by the night sweats and spontaneous sweating in the day, the dry mouth, alternation of heat and cold, some mental anxiety and the lack of energy. His immunity is low as shown by the chronic sweating and discharges and repeated cold sores as well as low energy. Symptoms also suggest ME but not confirmed at this point; no history of viral infection. He is also going through a stressful time as he is anxious to find work. Combined with this are symptoms of toxicity in the intestinal tract which is probably behind the elimination through the eyes and nose. The history of appendicitis and antibiotics is involved in this too. Treatment will be aimed at balancing his digestive system, supporting the endocrine and immune system to improve energy, relieving the superficial symptoms of discharges.

First treatment
Observations: client's feet felt very cool and clammy; his toes were like ice cubes. He was very stiff and couldn't relax.

Reflexes: none of his reflexes on the feet felt tender or sensitive. However he did report that when the appendix reflex area was touched he had a sensation in his right arm and when the diaphragm was touched in zone 3 he felt a warm sensation at the base of his back which spread right across. Feet feel thick and heavy to me. Remained cool throughout treatment.

Therapeutic strategy: whole foot treatment with special emphasis to endocrine system, immune system, kidneys, digestive, especially liver and upper respiratory system, eyes.

Recommendations: use camomile tea to rinse eyes every morning. Weekly treatments for six weeks, then reassess.

Second treatment
Response: on the day of the treatment he felt very good but on subsequent days his symptoms returned, his legs were aching and he continued to feel lethargic which he now says is his main problem.

Observations: feet were still cool but not so sweaty nor so cold today, warmed up with treatment.

Reflexes: still not sensitive, except the diaphragm, zone 2. Client is relaxing more into treatment.

Therapeutic strategy for next treatment: as previously.

Recommendation: adopt more simple diet, less meat and eat porridge for breakfast and a combination of rice and mung beans, cooked slowly together (kitcheree, see Chapter 11), as frequently as possible for dinner. This food is known to help in cases of weakness.

Third treatment
Response: herbal tea wash is helping the eyes on a daily basis. No change to nose and throat, still congested in the morning. Energy is still low especially in morning, legs are somewhat better.

Reflexes: gave whole foot treatment with special emphasis as previously to immune, endocrine and digestive systems. More sensitivity is showing in the feet. Right diaphragm reflex still tender and now the left adrenal reflex is a "bit tender". Feet are warming up with treatment.

Assessment: energy is beginning to flow better and organs and systems are responding. Slow but gradual improvement is beginning.

Therapeutic strategy: continue to emphasise the endocrine system, kidney-adrenals and digestive tract.

Recommendation: self-reflexology on liver, kidney and adrenal reflexes.

Fourth treatment
Response: rice and mung bean meals are helping a lot, feels more energy after eating. Felt better for two days after last treatment but is still lethargic in the morning though this has improved. Eyes have less discharge on some days, though some days it returns as badly.

Specific reflexes: diaphragm reflex still tender.

Assessment: feet are warming up with treatment though still cold when arrives. Client is relaxing more into treatment.

Fifth treatment
Response: client had a rough patch this week, eyes were worse again and legs heavy and felt lethargic. He had gone to London to take temporary work and have an interview, which however did not tire him out too much. He is continuing on the diet. His bowels are improving, are regular every day.

Reflexes: diaphragm reflex is still tender but less so. Right lung, zone 5 is tender. Left thyroid reflex is tender as is the clavicle lymph. Left foot sweated a little as right foot was worked on, but when it was worked on it warmed and sweating stopped.

Assessment: feet are not so cold at start, warm up and stay warm throughout treatment. Lymph reflexes are showing some life. Client was much more relaxed and his feet more flexible.

Therapeutic strategy: as previously.

Sixth treatment
Client had to stop treatments as he had found a job in London and was moving.

Summary
This was a complex case because although the client was young, he had experienced poor health for many years, since childhood, although nothing clinically serious was wrong. His immune system was weak and energy was low. However, improvement was beginning to show. Circulation had improved, he was more relaxed and symptoms had eased though were not completely clear. I believe this would have continued and gathered strength with more treatments and then he would be able to space out treatments to maintain what had been gained.

He had participated well in helping himself, adopting a better diet and working his own reflexes. Probably the securing of a job would remove much mental anxiety. His diet had improved and he was getting more high quality nourishment; his digestion had improved. His body had been strengthened enough that, if he could keep up these changes for himself, his health would keep on improving even though treatments had stopped. He was satisfied that he was getting better with the treatment.

Case 4
Mrs D, 56, happily married with three grown children

Complaint: Mrs D wanted to try reflexology to see if it would help her lose weight. Also she was having a lot of hot flushes, sweating heavily. She also gets a lot of pain in her breasts and stress incontinence with bladder and bowels (possible irritable bowel syndrome). Her legs hurt a lot at night, starting in early evening and often waking her up with pain.

Consultation revealed that the past ten or so years had been quite stressful as she had had to care a great deal for her elderly and ailing mother. Her mother had died about a year ago. About 25 years ago, after the birth of her two children she had developed varicose veins in her legs. Along with the present complaints of heat and sweating with leg cramps, incontinence, she has a bad taste in her mouth. She does a lot of self-help, putting her legs up in the evening, taking evening primrose oil and multivitamins. Her hobbies are community service. She gets little regular exercise, though walks a lot. Her sleep is poor as she wakes every two hours to pass urine and cannot resume sleep. Her mind worries in the night. Her legs often ache in the night, and she sometimes gets very tired. Three years ago she had flooding periods so underwent an endometrial re-section to remove the lining of the womb. This stopped the bleeding and periods altogether, but also weakened or traumatised the tissues so the incontinence began. She had always had heavy periods, but these had become worse over last ten years just as she was coping with her elderly parents (stress). Her diet includes a lot of fruit and vegetables, and meat daily. Her marriage is good one and she and her husband support one another.

Assessment: Mrs D is a very earnest and dutiful lady, always giving of herself to others. Finally she is taking some time to help herself and this is a good sign. She keeps meticulous daily records of her symptoms and what she eats. She is naturally of a heavy build but also has a tendency to put on weight, to have sluggish circulation, swollen ankles and be sedentary. There are also signs of excess heat, for example the heavy periods, blood imbalances causing clot, and of deficiency or irregularity, for example the stress of incontinence, hot flushes. She has been under tremendous stress over the past ten years. She is experiencing the effects of menopause but this is complicated by the traumas associated with the operation, and the years of stress.

First treatment
Observations: feet feel warm to client, cool to me. (She reports usually feeling warm due to the flushing.) Swelling below the ankles especially in the pelvic reflex areas, more than above and around the ankles themselves. Lower leg is oedematous and tense. Varicose veins are evident. Feet are stiff and inflexible to manipulation. Client keeps eyes open throughout treatment.

Reflexes: diaphragm is tender in both feet. Thyroid helper of left foot and right pituitary are tender. The transverse colon and small intestines are a little tender, and the tissue is thick around zone 1; the sigmoid colon reflex is very tender. The kidneys and adrenal glands and bladder are quite tender. The right breast area is tender as is the right uterus, chronic uterus/rectum and lymph/fallopian tube reflexes.

Assessment: these tender reflexes certainly reflect the areas of imbalance for this lady: the kidney-bladder, digestive and endocrine and reproductive areas.

Recommendations: weekly treatments for four weeks then reassess. Eat no or less meat in her diet to allow bowels to cleanse. Reduce or better, give up, tea and coffee, drink fennel tea. Take more regular exercise.

Second treatment
Response: client appalled that she actually put on weight. My response was that it would be better to concentrate on balancing the other ailments and then we could worry about that. For exercise I recommended yoga as this is helpful for digestion, muscle tone, as well as being relaxing and countering stress. She said she would think about it but wants to buy an exercise bike. Also had had terrible bowels all week, tender and diarrhoea. Other symptoms the same.

Specific reflexes: same reflexes tender as last treatment, now also liver shows tenderness. Gave extra attention to liver and gall bladder as well as reflexes in therapeutic strategy as above.

Assessment: client cannot relax, mind is very active monitoring everything, eyes stay open. Feet still stiff.

Recommendations: fennel tea, give up tea and coffee.

Third treatment
Response: some improvement in that she has slept better this week and has had no sweating; concentration is better. Other symptoms the same. She has bought an exercise bike to help circulation in her legs and weight; weight was stable. Has given up tea and coffee.

Specific reflexes: as before except the kidneys and left adrenals are no longer tender and the lower bowel and sigmoid colon less tender.

Therapeutic strategy: keep focusing on digestive tract and endocrine-lymph-reproductive system. Use more relaxation as client is still mentally and physically very tense.

Fourth treatment
Response: sleep is good now. Diarrhoea better and breasts not so sore. Had a bad gnawing pain in lower abdomen which she associated with the operation. She gets these occasionally.

Reflexes: the right bladder reflex was extremely tender, which it had not been before. Pituitary on both feet showing tenderness now. Kidney and left adrenals still not tender. Colon-sigmoid reflexes are clear now.

Assessment: the bladder reflex tenderness was a surprise and welcome as it shows energy is returning to this organ. Some gradual improvements continuing; still a long way to go. Patient still very tense. I feel there is a blockage here; she can't let go and allow the full effects of the treatment. She is controlling too much. She has not followed advice about yoga. She is so tense, understandably due to her experiences, but she is not aware of it.

Therapeutic strategy: continue to work on bladder reflex, with lots of relaxation; other reflexes as previously.

Recommendation: I felt that we had made some progress but that there was still a lot to do and recommended that we continue with weekly treatments. I suggested she eat daily a bowl of porridge for breakfast, to improve bowels, and nourish nervous system, build energy. I strongly urged her to do something to help her really relax. Perhaps a relaxation tape if she could not attend relaxation classes.

Fifth treatment
Response: bladder incontinence has improved a lot. Bowels are better, only in a.m. is there looseness. She feels her head is a lot calmer not so buzzing. She bought a relaxation tape and has been using it.

Observations: I noticed that Mrs D is now much more relaxed in herself. The relaxation tape seems to have helped her experience significant relaxation, perhaps for the first time in years. Also the improvement in the incontinence has eased her mind. Her body is now more relaxed as she receives treatment and her eyes close, while she is still aware and engaged in what is going on.

Specific reflexes: right thyroid helper, kidney and chronic uterus reflexes are tender. Uterus is tender on deep pressure. Swelling is still present around ankles but lower legs are softer, less tense. Groin lymph still tender. Other reflexes are less tender or clear.

Assessment: I feel a real breakthrough has been made as the client is so much more relaxed and the treatment is able to be more effective. Energy is beginning to flow more freely.

Sixth treatment

Response: incontinence is much improved, she is very glad about this. She has more colour in her cheeks and her friends have commented she does not look so tired. She is able to stay up a little later as she is not so dead tired in the evening. Legs are better but still ache badly some nights. She uses her relaxation tapes regularly and this helps a lot.

Specific reflexes: as before with little or no tenderness on left foot except in reproductive areas.

Recommendations and therapeutic strategy: continue as before, concentrate on glands and lymph and circulation to lessen oedema, ease cramps.

Summary

Mrs D continues to improve gradually, although some ailments return at times and she still has some very bad days. Probably if she could bring herself to let go of many of her responsibilities and give time just to herself, improvement would be even faster, but this is not possible at this time. She was able to have bi-weekly treatments and still maintain her progress. The lessening of the incontinence had been a tremendous boost. She had done a lot of self-help work which helped her a lot, and has become more self-aware and is able to relax and, most importantly, to know when she needs to relax and recuperate. Focus of treatment became the circulation and lymphatics to ease her legs and the endocrine glands to reduce flushes. She feels she has benefited tremendously from the treatments and continues to come regularly.

Observation: it would have been easy for both of us to get discouraged that not much significant improvement showed after the first four treatments and to have given up. I felt determined to keep trying with Mrs D and she was agreeable so we were able to continue and things began to gradually improve, especially when she changed within herself, let go of some of her control and tuned into her own inner needs more. She was growing into greater balance.

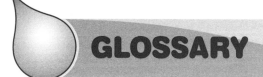
ABC – stands for Airway, Breathing and Circulation – the first things to check for in an unconscious casualty.

Accounts – the full and accurate record of all business transactions. This should be backed up with evidence, such as receipts for all purchases, chequebook stubs, bank statements, etc.

Active listening – listening with full attention to hear the other person's message and without concern to put over our own.

Adaptation – the means by which the body adapts, or changes in the face of a new, on-going, usually stressful, situation by making adjustments in its processes to ensure survival at optimal levels of functioning. Such adaptation can be short or longer lasting. If the latter, it may eventually lead to a deterioration in health.

AIDS – acquired immune deficiency syndrome, a condition, currently thought to be caused by the HIV virus, in which the body's immune system is so deficient or compromised that the body is highly susceptible to infections which can quickly become fatal.

Anatomical correspondences – the ways in which different parts of the body are anatomically related; that is, they have certain features in common though these are varied and not exactly the same. The curvature along the medial aspect of the toe mirrors or corresponds to the curvature of the spine. The shoulder is related to the hip because they both have appendages extending from them and are ball and socket joints.

Anterior – in front of; the front side.

Back-up reflex – a reflex that is worked to aid the functioning of a particular organ or system, because it is indirectly involved in its optimum health.

Being present – the therapist's ability and intention to maintain a state of awareness throughout the treatment session, thus acting as catalyst for the healing process.

Blocks to communication – pitfalls to be avoided in your relationship with clients. These include diagnosing, advising, and reassuring.

Breath awareness – breathing while listening consciously to the sound, and mentally following the flow of breath through its cycle so as to still the mind. It is used to centre the therapist before treatment and to clear the energy between treatments, or at any time to increase inner awareness.

Breathing-with-pressure technique – first a light and then gradually increasing pressure is applied to a single reflex as the client, and the therapist, consciously breathe deeply. It helps to remove the blockage, tenderness or congestion in the reflex point, and thus the corresponding part of the body.

Business plan – the strategy setting out how the business will be set up and funds obtained for any needed expenditure; usually required by banks before they will agree a loan.

Carpal bones – eight small bones in the wrist.

Case history – the record of a client's personal details taken at the first appointment and kept up to date. *See also* Treatment record.

Cashflow forecast – a forecast of how much cash a business is likely to generate in a specified period in the future. The cashflow itself is the difference between outgoings and receipts over a given period.

Catalyst – a substance or action that influences a process, without itself being changed.

Cautions – self-warnings, i.e. when certain disease conditions call for extra care or expertise on the part of the reflexologist because they are so serious for the client. The reflexologist may choose or not choose to give treatment depending on her level of training and experience and she may prefer to consult the client's physician before proceeding.

Closing – the ending of the reflexology treatment session when the treatment is discussed with the client, and recommendations or advice are given.

Code of ethics – standards of conduct, often set down by professional organisations for their members. Includes such matters as working within the limits of training and confidentiality. Also often known as Code of Conduct or Code of Practice.

Cross reflexes – areas of the body which are anatomically, and therefore energetically, related and which can be worked when it is not possible to work the related counterpart due to disease or injury. For example, the elbow is the cross reflex for the knee.

Crystals – areas of tissue under the skin that feel hard, gritty, sandy, congested or tense to the touch. They may or may not be tender when touched.

Distal – at a distance from the centre; for example the leg is distal to the heart, the toe is distal to the ankle.

Door opener – a brief statement indicating that you are available to listen. For example: 'You seem a bit tense today . . .'

Dorsal – the back side, the top side of the foot/hand; opposite to the plantar/palmar side.

Dynamic – characterised by vital energy, power; energised and capable of activity.

Eliciting – evoking information by gentle means; bringing into the light, into awareness.

Elimination channels – the five means by which the body rids itself of waste: the colon, skin, lungs, kidneys and lymph.

Encouraging statement – a brief verbal expression designed to encourage a client to start, or continue, talking. They show that the listener is present and that the speaker's world-view is valid. The most obvious example is 'Mm – hmm'. Some others are: 'I see, go on . . .'; 'Then . . . ?' 'Tell me more . . .'; 'Really?'

Healing crisis or achievement – a process of healing which the body undertakes to balance itself or when it is ready to throw out the remnants of a disease condition. Although it brings its discomforts as the elimination of wastes and toxins occurs, it is really a positive sign of the return of higher vitality to the body.

Hemispheres – the two halves of the brain, or cerebrum. Each is recognised to be responsible for certain activities, although in practice both are always involved to a certain extent. *See also* Left and right brain.

HIV – Human Immunodeficiency Virus, thought to be responsible for AIDS.

Holistic – an approach to health care which recognises that not just physical factors, such as pathogens or trauma, but also the interrelationships between mind, body and spirit are involved in the creation of disease and recovery of health. Understanding and treating the whole person.

Homeostasis – the body's feedback mechanism for maintaining optimum levels of gases, ions, water and nutrients as well as pressure and temperature to ensure its health.

Hook-in-back-up technique the thumb is flexed and presses down into the reflex point and then drags back towards the middle of the hand. It is found to be more effective for some points such as the pituitary, pineal and ileo-caecal valve reflexes.

Hospice – a special hospital for terminally ill patients, where palliative treatment and loving care is given, but not curative medical interventions.

Inflammation – a local fever. Characterised by heat, swelling, redness and pain.

Integrity – from the Latin for wholeness; inner and outer honesty, and high ethical standing.

Intention – that aspect of treatment in which the therapist's mind and energy is directed toward the goal of working with the natural healing energy without force; it is a positive but passive state, being open to change but allowing the body to change when it is ready.

Intuition – that aspect of the mental faculties which relies on non-logical modes of understanding beyond mere reason or physical perception.

Landmarks – physical features of the foot and hand which can be used to demarcate an area or orient the reflexologist to a particular reflex or area, for example the toes, the fifth metatarsal/carpal prominence, the heel line, the diaphragm line, the tendon, the ankle.

Lateral – the outer side, the side of the foot where the arm and shoulder reflexes are located.

Left and right brain – the left hemisphere of the cerebrtal cortex is thought to be responsible for logical, analytic thinking; the right hemisphere for intuition and creative thought.

Light-holding technique – reflex technique in which only a very light pressure is applied to a reflex and held stationary for a few moments, while the practitioner maintains presence. It works somewhat subtly, waiting patiently for the body to respond to the energy exchange. Response can be gauged by changes in temperature, tension or congestion, as well as by the therapist's experience.

Limits of training – the responsibilty a therapist has to recognise when a client has needs which cannot be met by her skills; knowing when to refer a client to another practitioner. An essential aspect of professional integrity.

Major areas – the main general areas of the foot corresponding to the larger areas of the body – the head, chest, abdominal, and pelvic regions.

Medial – the middle, the side of the feet where the spine reflex is located.

Open questions – questions phrased in such a way as to encourage the client to share more detail; the opposite of closed questions which require only a yes or no answer.

Paraphrasing – a useful technique allowing the therapist to cut through clutter to try to get to the heart of what the client is saying.

Peri-natal – the period around the birth, just before and just after.

Personal development – the obligation, shared by all holistic practitioners, to take responsibilty for the health not only of their own body, but of their mind and spirit. The on-going development of self-awareness as an integral part of the practitioner's life.

Pivoting technique (or pivoting-on-a-point) – a technique in which the thumb is placed fixedly on a reflex and the support hand moves the foot onto and around that point.

Plantar – the sole side of the foot.

Pollex – the thumb.

Posterior – behind, the back side.

Post-natal – the period immediately after birth and lasting a week or two.

Presence – a state of mindfulness and inner awareness which is – as much as possible – free of concern for either past or future and fully open to or accepting present experience without prejudging what occurs.

Professional development – the obligation of the reflexologist to keep skills up to date and to continue to develop skills by engaging in further training on a regular basis.

Proximal – opposite of *distal*. Situated towards the centre of the body. The toe is at the distal end of the foot, while ankle and heel are the proximal ends.

Recovery position – the position into which an unconscious casualty is placed.

Referral – when a client's needs are beyond the scope of a reflexologist's training or expertise, the reflexologist will have no hesitation in advising, or referring, the client to other profesionals. *See also* Limits of training.

Relapse – moving backwards to a previous negative state after having progressed some way out of it.

Right brain – *see* Left brain.

Sciatic loop – the area on the foot, from behind the ankles and around under the heel, which helps sciatic problems.

Self-esteem – the fundamental security in one's own value which allows a person to give love and enter into positive relationships with other human beings. Not to be confused with egoism.

Stages of disease – the stages through which the body's healthy functioning is compromised so that disease can appear. They are: acute sub-acute, chronic, degenerative.

Stress response – the body's natural response to stress of any kind through a sequence of nervous and hormonal changes that affect the mind, emotions, physical tissues and organs.

Summarising – the therapist brings together the key points raised by the client. A particularly useful technique in the initial consultation as it provides an overview of the issues and a clue to where your work might begin.

Support holds – methods of holding and supporting the client's foot or hand so that the therapist's working hand can accomplish its tasks as efficiently and comfortably as possible.

Synergy – the concept that the whole is greater than merely the sum of its parts, that when the different parts act in concert a greater, different energy is created than can be attributed to any one of them singly.

Tax return – the form supplied by the Inland Revenue on which you record your earnings for the past year, any capital gains and your net profit.

Tender reflexes – areas on the feet and hands which feel tender or painful to the client when given reflex pressure.

Therapeutic space – an area of time and place where the client enjoys comfort, security and calm so that mind and body can become deeply relaxed and thus more open to healing energy from within.

Thyroid helper – the reflex that is located close to the thyroid reflex in zone 1 of the plantar chest area. It is beneficial to work this reflex whenever there are thyroid problems.

Transference – projecting onto another person responsibility for one's happiness, or equally, for one's negative situation.

Treatment record – the continuation of a case history into the present treatment.

VAT – Value Added Tax is charged to most goods and services. A reflexologist, as provider of a service, may be liable once the turnover of her business reaches a specified limit, currently £54,000.

Vital force – the power that creates and sustains the universe and every thing and every creature in it. The energy that gives and maintains life.

Vulnerability – the state of being open to attack or being taken advantage of.

Walking technique – the efficient use of the finger or thumb to give pressure to reflexes in close sequence while moving rhythmically over the foot or hand.

Zone – an area of the body affected by the flow of an energy line.

RESOURCES AND FURTHER READING

Further reading

Balch, James F. and Balch, Phyllis A. *Prescription for Nutritional Healing.* Avery Publishing, New York. 2001.

Ball, John. *Understanding Disease.* C.W. Daniel Ltd, Saffron Walden, Essex. 1990.

Ballentine, Rudolph. *Diet and Nutrition.* Himalyan Press, Honesdale, Pennsylvania. 1978.

Benson, H. *The Relaxation Response.* Avon, London. 1976.

Brennan, Barbara Ann. *Hands of Light.* Bantam Books, London. 1988.

Byers, Dwight. *Better Health with Foot Reflexology.* Ingham Publishing, Florida. 1994.

Coghill, Roger. 'Medicine for the New Millennium' in *International Journal of Alternative and Complementary Medicine*, Dec. 1998 (pgs. 19-20).

Cousins, Norman. *Anatomy of an Illness As Perceived by the Patient.* Norton, New York. 1979.

Dalton, Katharina and Holton, Wendy. *Depression after Childbirth, How to Recognize, Treat and Prevent Postnatal Depression.* Oxford University Press. 1996.

Diamond, Harvey and Diamond, Marilyn. *Fit for Life*, Bantam Books, London. 1987.

Featherstone, Cornelia and Forsythe, Lori. *Medical Marriage: The New Partnership.* Findhorn Press, London. 1997.

Hippocrates. *Works* W.H.S. Jones, translator. Loeb Classical Library, Harvard University Press. 1923.

Ingham, Eunice. *Stories the Feet Can Tell* and *Stories the Feet Have Told.* Ingham Publishing, Florida. *1992.*

Institute of Noetic Sciences with William Poole. *The Heart of Healing.* Turner Publishing, Atlanta. 1993.

Issel, Christine. *Reflexology, Art, Science and History.* New Frontier Publishing, Sacramento, California. 1990.

Kaptchuk, Ted. *The Web That Has No Weaver*, revised edition. Rider, London. 2000.

Kreiger, Dolores. *The Therapeutic Touch, How to Use Your Hand to Help or to Heal.* Prentice-Hall, Englewood Cliffs. New Jersey. 1982.

Kunz, Barbara and Kunz, Kevin. *The Complete Guide to Foot Reflexology.* Thorsens/Harper Collins, London. 1984.

Lad, Vasant. *Ayurved: The Science of Self-Healing*. Lotus Press, Wilmot, WI. 1984.

Mernagh-Ward, Dawn and Cartwright, Jennifer. *Good Practice in Salon Management*. Stanley Thornes (Publishers) Ltd, Cheltenham. 1997.

Mitchell, Annie. Lecturer in Psychology and Complementary Health Studies, Exeter University: 'The Therapeutic Relationship in Health Care: towards a model of the process of treatment'. *Journal of Interprofessional Care*, Vol. 9, No.1. 1995.

Mitchell, A. and Cormak, M. *The Therapeutic Relationship in Health Care*. Churchill Livingstone, London. 1998.

Montague, Ashley. *Touching: The Human Significance of the Skin*. Harper Collins, London. 1986.

Morrison, Judith. *The Book of Ayurveda*. Gaia Books, London. 1994.

Murray, Michael and Pizorno, Joseph. *Encyclopedia of Natural Medicine*. Little Brown & Company, New York and London. 1990.

Newman-Turner, Roger. *Naturopathic Medicine*. Thorsens/Harper Collins, London. 1990.

Norman, Laura. *The Reflexology Handbook*. Piatkus Publishers Ltd, London. 1989.

Ornish, Dean. *Dr Dean Ornish's Program for Reversing Heart Disease*. Ivy Books, New York. 1996.

Oschman, James L. *Energy Medicine: The Scientific Basis*. Churchill Livingstone, London. 2000.

Page, Christine. *Frontiers of Health*, C.W. Daniel, Saffron Walden. 2000.

Pietroni, Patrick. *The Greening of Medicine*. Victor Gollancz, London. 1990.

Pitman, Vicki. *Herbal Remedies*. Chrysalis Books, London. 2001.

Sams, Jamie. *Earth Medicine – Ancestors' Ways of Harmony for Many Moons*. Harper, San Francisco, 1994.

Selye, Hans. *The Stress of Life*. McGraw-Hill, London. 1990.

St. Pierre, Gaston and Shapiro, Debbie. *The Metamorphic Technique*. Element Books, Shaftesbury, Dorset. 1982.

Stormer, Chris. *Reflexology – The Definitive Guide*. Hodder & Stoughton Educational, London. 1995.

Wagner, Franz. *Reflex Zone Massage*. Thorsens/Harper Collins. 1987.

Walker, Kristine. *Hand Reflexology: A textbook for students*. Quay Books, Mark Allen Publishing Group, Snow Hill, Dinton, Wiltshire SP3 5HN. 1996.

Useful addresses and websites

The Association of
Reflexologists
27 Old Gloucester Street
London
WC1N 3XX
www.aor.org.uk

British Complementary
Medicine Association
Soar Lane, Leicester
LE3 5DE
or – BCMA
PO Box 2074
Seaford
BN25 1HQ
www.bcma.co.uk

British Reflexology
Association
Monks Orchard
Witbourne
Worcester
WR6 5RB
www.britreflex.co.uk

Edward Bach Centre
(sales of Bach flower remedies
and related publications)
Mount Vernon
Sotwell
OX10 0PZ
www.bachcentre.com

The Gateway Clinic
(holistic approach to
substance abuse and
HIV-AIDS)
Lambeth Healthcare
NHS Trust
108 Landor Road
Stockwell
London
SW9 9NT

Holistic Association of
Reflexologists
The Holistic Healing Centre
92 Sheering Road
Old Harlow
CM17 0JW
www.footreflexology.com

House of Lords Select Committee
on Science and Technology's
Report on Complementary and
Alternative Medicine
Price: £15.50
Available from
The Stationery Office,
PO Box 29,
Norwich
NR3 1GN
email: bookorders@theso.co.uk
or view it on the government
website at: www.parliament.
the-stationery-office.co.uk

International Council for
Reflexology
www.ict-reflexology.org

International Federation of
Reflexologists
78 Eldridge Road
Croydon
CR10 1EF
www.reflexology-ifr.com

International Institute of
Reflexology
5650 First Avenue North
PO Box 12642
St Petersburg
Florida
33733–2642
USA
www.reflexology-usa.net

International Institute of
Reflexology (UK)
The Reflexology Centre
32 Priory Road
Portbury
Bristol
BS20 9TH
or – 255 Turleigh
Bradford-on-Avon
BA15 2HG
www.reflexology-uk.co.uk

International Therapy
Examination Council
10–11 Heathfield Terrace
Chiswick
London
W4 4JE
www.itecworld.co.uk
Irish Reflexologists' Institute
The Secretary
4 Ruskin Park
Lisburn
Co. Antrim
email: www.reflexology.ie

Reflexology Academy
of Southern Africa
PO Box 1280,
Rivonia 2128
Gauteng
Republic of South Africa
Reflexology Association of America
4012 S. Rainbow Boulevard
Box K585
Las Vegas
Nevada 89103–2059
USA
www.reflexology-usa.org

Reflexology in Europe
Network
www.reflexeurope.org
Reflexology Sales
(sales of books, charts, etc.
on reflexology)
Unit 4, Willow Farm
Allwood Green
Rickinghall
Diss
Norfolk
IP22 1LT

Scottish Institute of
Reflexology
17 Cainwell Avenue
Mastrick
Aberdeen
AB16 5SH
www.scottishreflexology.org

Society of Reflexologists
39 Prestbury Road
Cheltenham
GL52 2PT

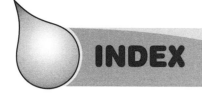

INDEX

Page references in **bold** indicate figures or tables